To Gloria

Living Cancer Living Truth

Love and best wishes

Lesley

Visit www.booksurge.com to order additional copies.

Living Cancer
Living Truth

Lesley Moore

2007

Living Cancer Living Truth

For my parents

"When I said that no one can honestly claim to know the cure for breast cancer, I was telling a half-truth. If a patient could promote the healing process from within, that would be *the* cure for cancer."

Deepak Chopra in *Quantum Healing: Exploring the Frontiers of Mind/Body Medicine*

Preface

You can guess my reaction to cancer. I was shocked and tearful. I couldn't take everything in. I couldn't understand how it had happened to me. I was scared of what would happen to my body. I was afraid I was going to die.

What will surprise you is what came next. Half an hour after the diagnosis I was euphoric, and the nine months after that taking me through a mastectomy and chemotherapy were, until recently, the very best months of my life.

Coming out of cancer my goal has been to create a life where I can be as alive and as free as I was with cancer. I want to experience life as I did with cancer. I want to feel about life the way that I did with cancer.

Now, five years on, my life is richer and more wonderful than it has ever been and more magical than I thought possible. And I owe this all to cancer—or rather to my body—and what it has taught me about life, health, faith and truth.

Anyone with cancer *can* embrace the disease and experience it positively. For me it just happened that way; most people are not so fortunate. This book is for you.

PART ONE

I

Cancer gave me back my life and showed me how to live. Cancer was my salvation. I definitely needed saving, why I'll explain in a minute. More important than that is for you to know that I *knew* I needed to be saved and desperately wanted to be. I also knew that gifts often come in unlikely packages and that I'd know it—whatever 'it' was—when I saw it. You see I'd been there before. Not a major illness—something my mum said when I told her I had cancer was, "but Lesley, you're *never* ill!"—but another life-changing event that had a completely unexpected and thrilling effect on me.'

My husband left in October 1998 after we'd been married seven years. Three months earlier I'd given up my full-time, well-paid job of seven years to be a full-time mum supported by him, when before that he'd been more or less supported by me. I'd not seen this coming. I didn't want my husband to leave, I didn't want my marriage to end and I certainly didn't want to be solely responsible for a small child and a mortgage. As a result I was upset when he said he was going to leave but this feeling was soon replaced by another.

I was doing a 'change your life' course at the time—not the first or the last—and once a week I called my coach to talk about my issues. It was because of a conversation with my coach—don't ask me what he said, I can't remember and don't worry, it really isn't important to this story—that, for the first time in my marriage, indeed the whole relationship, I listened to my husband. I mean *really* listened. Before then I'd heard what he said some of the time, but I'd never listened with my *whole being*.

If that sounds a bit 'new age' to you, I guess it is. So you may as well find out now, before you get too hooked, that there's more of that to come. Just wait until you get to page...Sorry! Just a little joke I couldn't resist. Did you really think I'd send you off into the depths of the book? I couldn't, because I need your attention—all of it—here and now. Although I'm being light-hearted this is a serious issue. It's something you need to think hard about.

Will my new age tendencies put you off this book?
Indeed, will anything about me put you off this book?

Maybe you don't like my chatty style. Maybe you don't like my tone. Maybe, because I reacted to cancer as I did, you think I'm deranged. Or maybe it's worse than that. Maybe you already *hate* me because I enjoyed cancer when it's the worst thing that's happened to you, shattering your world and making you feel completely lost and helpless; so desperate, in fact, that you're reading this book even though you think I'm a complete jerk!

Some of you won't like me and/or my writing style while to others I'll be inspirational, but to those of you that are having problems with me and/or the book I want to say this: Bear with me. It takes time to get to know and trust somebody, especially when her outlook and experiences are so different from your own, and it takes even longer if there are things about her you don't like—things that get your barriers up. Yes, I am new agey. Yes, I'm chatty and make bad jokes. Yes, I have a very different take on cancer—but that's the point! You're reading this book *because* I have something different to say. Please don't let what I'm saying or how I say it put you off now, at the very beginning.

Think about it for a minute. What's the worst that can happen? You get to the end of the book and think, "what rubbish, what a waste of the cover price and a few days". But what's the best that can happen? You can't even begin to imagine. You already have cancer. You're already living the nightmare. Please let me show you how to turn that around. It's all I want—I want nothing *from* you—I simply want to show you there is another way.

What do I mean when I say I listened to my husband with my whole being? Put your hand on your stomach, in the space between your belly button and your heart, and feel what it's like to have your hand there. That's where I heard him. Not in my head, but there. And it was as if I could feel what he was saying, not in an emotional 'my husband's dumping me, oh woe is me!' kind of way, but in a very simple way. I could feel what he was saying inside my body. Everywhere inside. Inside my arms, in my legs and in my torso. It was a very subtle sensation and it had no emotional content. In fact, trying to describe this feeling to you, I think it was that—the sensation associated with the complete absence of emotion and indeed anything else. It was the sensation associated with nothing. And accompanying this sensation was an incredible awareness and clarity and an amazing sense of silence and peace.

It was the peace and silence that struck me as I listened to him. It wasn't that we'd spent the whole time arguing— ours had been a relationship characterised by silence, certainly towards the end anyhow. No, the silence wasn't to do with him, or with our relationship, but with me. It was to do with the listening. To understand what I mean by that you need to put yourself inside my head as it used to be. How was it? Full. I mean *really* full. So full, I don't know how I fitted it all in. If I had to get that much in my head now I'd need g-cramps on my skull to hold it together! But back then I didn't notice. I had no idea how full my head was. Yes, there were pointers, but I ignored them.

"You think too much!" my husband would say.

To which I would reply, inside my head of course: "You don't think enough!" or "You don't know what you're talking about!" My head was full of stuff I knew and one thing I knew for certain was that I knew better than him! No surprise then that I was out of the habit, if I'd ever been in it, of listening to him. Everything he said went through my 'I know better than you' filter and if he said something I didn't like or didn't agree with, I paid no attention to him. Even when he said, "this is important to me," if I didn't think the issue was important I'd do nothing about it. I wonder why he left me?!

Of course I didn't know I was a know-it-all—ha! just got the irony of that one—it was simply something I'd become. It crept up on me slowly and took me over, like lots and lots of other stuff. The main problem wasn't the stuff that inhabited my brain though, but my brain itself. I have a good brain—part of the reason I was such a know-it-all was that I took what the education system said to heart, i.e. academically bright equals top of the tree, and it didn't even cross my mind to listen to those poor souls in the branches below—and I learned to use my brain very effectively. So effectively, in fact, that it replaced everything else. By the time my husband finally left—he'd tried to leave before but I'd always talked him out of it; I mean, I knew he didn't really *want* to leave, did he?!—virtually all of my life was controlled by my brain. Everything I thought, said and did was the product of my enormous processor of a brain and its constant hum was, unknowingly, the background noise of my life.

So when I finally listened to my husband—not through my know-it-all filter; indeed not through my brain at all—the silence was astounding. The noise stopped. I stopped. And time stood still. Thus when he spoke, his words had space to be and the peace came just from the experience of listening; from putting myself completely to one side and listening to what another human being had to say. What did he say? "I want to leave. I'm going to leave. And nothing you can say or do will change my mind"—or something like that. Exactly what he said is not important. The point is that I listened and I heard him. I heard the truth in his words and I knew I had to let him go. Whatever I thought or felt was irrelevant. I had to let him go.

At some level the act of listening was the same as flicking a switch. Before I listened my brain was fully on and my body and life were fully off. The listening activated my body and kick-started my life again, relegating my mind to what I consider to be its rightful place—remembering what to buy from the shops, how to program the video and when to pay the bills. When I listened to my husband I knew I had no choice but to let him go. Having heard him—really heard him—I knew that to try to make him stay would have been to deny the truth. It would have meant deluding myself that there was something to save in the relationship, something worth fighting for, and I knew from what he'd said that this was not the case.

And in that moment when I put myself completely aside to listen to him, I felt what it's like to embrace truth in the absence of oneself. It's exhilarating! Think watching a theme park ride on TV and then being on that roller coaster. Can you imagine what that's like? To in an instant feel alive having been in suspended animation for such a long, long time?

It's amazing.
It's incredible.
It's life changing.

It was like that when I embraced the truth of my husband leaving. It was like that when I embraced the truth of cancer. The difference was with cancer, I was *not* going to let that feeling go.

2

People are funny. They only see what they want to see. Yes, I had no husband or job, a mortgage to pay and a toddler to look after—but I was happy. It was OK. I knew it would be all right.

It's the knowing that's important. It makes all the difference. I'm not sure where it comes from but does that matter? Just because I can't explain why or how, does that make it less real, less useful or less valid? The thing about knowing is that's what it is: *knowing*. You don't know why you know, or how you know, you just know. You know it in your body—in that place between your belly button and your heart. Put your hand there again—there, that's where you know. And it's so different from being a know-it-all, because to *know* you don't need to know anything at all!

Know-it-alls know lots of stuff—take it from me, I was one for most of my life. We know the way the world works: we've spent a long time analysing it. We know how people work: we've spent a long time figuring them out. We know where we're headed in life. Why wouldn't we? We know everything! Knowing isn't like that. Knowing is different. When you *know*, you don't know anything apart from the fact that you know.

I knew when my husband left that it would be OK. That this was a turning point in my life and that everything would be better for it. And it was the same with cancer. I knew this was the thing I'd been waiting for: that gift in the unlikely package. I knew cancer would turn my life around and make it better. And more than anything else,

I knew I must not let the opportunity go to waste as I'd done before.

So who are those funny people? Everybody apart from you and if you're lucky a handful of loyal and trusting friends. What's funny about them? Mmm...how can I put this? There's no easy way to do it, so I'll just say it. Most people are not interested in the truth. Most people do not have your best interests at heart. Most people want things to be the way they want things to be: the way that agrees with what they know. Yes, most people are know-it-alls. They know how to react when your husband leaves, you've a mortgage to pay, no job and a small child to look after. There is only one way *to* react. You are upset, you blame him and of course it's his fault. You feel hopeless, you feel helpless and your life falls apart. But very very slowly, you... pick up the pieces, and...when the time is right...after a suitable period of grief...you pull yourself together and get on with it.

But more than that, they know how you shouldn't react. You shouldn't be happy. You shouldn't say, "my husband leaving has given me access to my truth". You shouldn't say, "everything will be OK, I know it will". They don't want things you can't explain; they want answers to their questions. How will it be OK? How can this be true? How will you pay the mortgage? How will you work with a small child? And some people know so much they don't even need to ask questions. They know so much, they know exactly how it is. How awful it is that you gave up your job only three months ago. What a bastard he is for leaving. How terrible the situation is. And these people also know that when you do not react as you should—indeed, when you react exactly as you should not—something is wrong. And because these people know everything, they know that what is wrong is you.

I feel I need a parable, but I don't have one—or maybe this whole story is a parable? What I'm looking for is a way to explain what happened next, but maybe that's blindingly obvious and what I'm trying to find is a way of making it interesting when it's not. So I'd better get on with it. After my husband left I let the know-it-alls get the better of me—and weren't they happy about it! They'd known they were right all along! They knew I'd reacted as I did because I was in shock, that the feeling of euphoria couldn't last forever because it wasn't real, and that after a while I'd come down to earth with a bump. And that I did but not with a bump—if it had happened that way I'd have noticed and could have done something about it, but it wasn't like that. As with all the most dangerous things in life it crept up on me slowly and silently. Which is why, by the time my body gave me cancer, I needed saving—again!

3

Now is a good time to tell you that my body gave me cancer for that reason: to save me. Or rather, to save me from myself. Key questions are therefore:

Why did I need saving?
Why did it take my body to do it?
Why couldn't I figure it out by myself? (I tried that.)
Or read some books? (I read loads.)
Or get someone else to help me? (I did that too.)

I needed my body to save me because I couldn't be saved in any other way. The thing I needed saving from was too big, it had too big a hold on me and it didn't want to let go.

"But wait a minute!" I hear you cry. "Didn't you say the thing you needed saving from was yourself? And now you're telling me that this thing, i.e. you, had too big a hold on *you* and wouldn't go without a fight. What are you talking about? It doesn't make sense!"

Ah, yes. That's not going to be easy to explain, is it? Not in a way that gives you a bodily understanding of what I'm talking about. It's no good me telling you how it is, that won't do at all. You need to understand not with your head, but with your body. You need to begin to *know*. So with apologies and thanks to Clarissa Pinkola Estés, author of *Women Who Run with the Wolves*, I feel a fairy tale coming on.

Once upon a time there was a little girl. She was born into a village of giants but, little did anyone know, she was not a giant at all. Her parents believed she was a giant, as did everyone in the village. It did not cross their minds that she might be something other than a giant, for they did not know that such creatures existed.

The day that she was born there was great rejoicing. The mother and father were very happy. They had wanted a child for some time and were very proud of their little daughter. As was the giants' tradition, all the people in the village came to visit, to honour the parents and their baby. With them they brought many gifts, all perfect for a baby giant. These gifts were not the gifts that humans give. There were no presents wrapped in brightly coloured paper. There were no toys or books. Instead, with him or her, each giant brought an 'understanding'—the thing that, to each of them, was the most important thing for a giant to know.

These understandings had a sacred place in the world of the giants and, in giving the gift, each giant believed that he or she was bestowing upon the little girl great knowledge and wisdom and thus ensuring her continued good health and future happiness. And, of course, this would have been the case had the little girl been a giant but, as we know, she was not one at all. As soon as they were given the gifts started to work on the little girl, and because they were so powerful the little girl forgot, before she had time to tell anyone, that she was not a giant. Without the knowledge that she was not a giant the little girl had no choice but to become one. How could she become anything else when giants did not know that creatures other than giants existed?

Thanks to the gifts given by the giants the little girl grew to be knowledgeable and wise in the ways of the giants. She worked hard in the ways that giants should work hard. She took pleasure in the things that giants should take pleasure in. She led, as far as the other giants were concerned, an exemplary existence. She was a giant to be proud of, a tribute to her parents and to the villagers who had taken such care in choosing their gifts.

One day the little girl was collecting wood in the forest when she heard a voice from behind a tree.

"Little girl, little girl, do you know my name?"

The little girl was startled by the voice and afraid, and ran back home as fast as her legs would carry her. Wondering why the little girl was back so soon and without any wood her parents asked what had happened. The little girl told them of the voice and asked who had spoken. Her mother and father did not know but said it was probably one of the other children from the village and that the little girl should not worry.

The next day the little girl went back into the forest to gather wood and as before the voice came from behind a tree.

"Little girl, little girl, do you know my name?"

Again the little girl was frightened, for the voice did not sound like any voice she had heard before, and again she ran back home as fast as her legs would carry her. Her parents were angry to see her home so soon, again without any wood, and asked what had happened. Again the little girl told them about the voice and again her parents told her that it was just a child from the village and to forget it had happened.

The next day the little girl went back into the forest to gather wood and again the voice came from behind a tree.

"Little girl, little girl, do you know my name?"

But this time, before the little girl had time to run, a shot rang out in the forest and she heard something fall behind the tree where the voice had come from. More interested now than afraid the little girl walked over to the tree and looked behind it. There lay another little girl, quite unlike any person she had seen before.

The child had been injured by the shot but was still alive and because she was too big to move the little girl rushed back to her parents' house to get help. The mother and father followed the little girl into the forest but when they saw the other child they were afraid. This girl was not like anybody they had seen before. Nothing about her was familiar and they were afraid to help her. Turning their backs on the injured child the mother and father started for home, telling the little girl to come with them. She refused. Nothing they said would change the little girl's mind and because she was holding the hand of the other girl they were afraid to take her with them.

Word spread around the village of the strange child in the forest and the actions of the little girl. One by one the villagers came to talk to the little girl and ask her to come home. They talked of the village and how her parents missed her. They talked of her friends and the games they could play together. They talked of the way of the giants and how important it was for the little girl to follow the way. One by one they came but nothing the villagers said made any difference. Still the little girl stayed with the child, holding her hand and keeping her warm.

The little girl stayed in the forest for many days. But in all this time, the injured child never spoke to her or woke from the sleep into which she had fallen. Then one day without warning, the child opened her eyes, smiled at the little girl, said "thank you", kissed her on the cheek and ran away. And what did the little girl do? She ran after her.

For now you'll have to take that for what it is: a fairy tale written by me in an attempt to explain something I don't yet understand. But to help you accept this—both the fairy tale and the approach, and to stop you throwing your hands up in horror and this book in the bin!—I'll share with you the words of the storytelling master herself, Clarissa Pinkola Estés. These are taken from her book *Women Who Run with the Wolves,* save for the words in brackets which have been added by me.

"Fairy tales, myths and stories provide understandings which sharpen our sight so that we can pick out and pick up the path left by our wildish nature [our lost selves]."

"The instruction found in story reassures us that the path has not run out, but leads women [and men] deeper, and more deeply still, into their own knowing."

"Stories are medicine."
"Stories set the inner life into motion."
"Stories...lead us back to our own real lives."

4

This book is a story. It's the story of my life and how cancer transformed both it and me. It's written as a story is told in the oral tradition, i.e. starting at the beginning and working through to the end, and it's born of my creativity and intuition.

I've not planned out this book. I don't know what path it will take and what twists and turns it will make in getting to the end. And that, contrary to what the intellect may say, is a good thing. It allows me, through my writing, to draw on things I do not yet understand and things I do not yet know. And so this book works in the same way as everything else that's worked in my life. That's life after my husband left but before the know-it-alls got to me, life after I was diagnosed with cancer, and life after I sold my house to write this book. In that, I don't know exactly what I'm doing, or how I'm going to get to the end of it, or how it's going to be all right, but that's exactly what it *is* going to be—all right. I know it is.

I know because I feel it in my body and I trust this feeling more than I trust anything else in this life. I use this—and this alone—to guide me. And it's this I want you to have access to. I want you to know which way to turn in life and to have such faith in that knowing that it allows you to do the most incredible things. Things that astound and confound others and which are, in their eyes, either extraordinarily brave or extraordinarily stupid but that to you are nothing. Why? Because they are simply things you must do, because to not do them would be unthinkable.

What's required?
Listen to what your body wants and do it.

I know that sounds too simple and too good to be true but it's not. The problem comes in hearing your body above the noise of what *you* do and do not want to do—but I'll deal with that later. Now I want to show you how listening to my body helped me write this book. When I finished the last chapter I didn't know what to write next and instead of the next line, what kept coming to mind were the work-related files I'd amassed after my husband left and I set up business from home. Archiving these files is something I could have done at any point over the past year (when I closed down my consultancy business to focus on this book) but for one reason and another have avoided doing.

These damned files are on my mind because I'm having new software installed on my computer and I know there's no need for them to be on my hard disc, taking up room and reminding me of the old life I'm happy to have left behind. All week these files have popped into my head in the nagging way that issues appear when you know you've to attend to them but don't want to. Those thoughts appear in quite a violent way, don't they? They force their way in from the side. They arrive abruptly and angrily. They oust whatever else is there. When the files made themselves known today, however, they did so very softly and gently, with an awareness of them blossoming within my body like a flower. And partly because they came that way, and partly because I finally wanted to, I archived those files to disc.

And now to the point of the story. It was through the archive process that I saw something I need to say in this book, i.e. I was given part of the puzzle. The archiving and verification took only ten minutes each—no time at all;

this was a task I could have fitted into almost any day. But it's not how long it took me to do the task that's of interest here but how long it took to be *ready* to do it—over a year. Once I was ready I did it no problem, but before then it seemed an impossible task.

And this takes me forward to cancer. If you've been wondering how I saw the upside of cancer so quickly—after half-an-hour as it says in the Preface—I was ready to do it, that's all. And it is as simple as that—a case of being ready—but it's also the huge effort that goes into being ready that is important to grasp and appreciate. Think of a man winning a gold medal at the Olympic Games—I think he also does this simply because he's ready to, because it is his time. But both you and I know that to win an Olympic gold that man could not sit around for months on end then turn up at the track and win. No, he has to put in lots of hard work over many years in order to achieve it. Indeed to be a top-class athlete, he has to dedicate his whole life to the sport, setting aside other things in order to achieve his goal.

Being ready isn't something that just happens—it takes effort—and the bigger the prize the more effort you have to put in. Being ready to catch a bus simply requires that you get yourself to the bus stop in time with enough money in your pocket to pay the fare. But being ready to win Olympic gold—or to accept and embrace cancer and actually enjoy the experience—that takes a lot more effort. Don't let yourself be put off by this—it doesn't mean it can't be done by you. Let's be clear: I'm talking about the positive experience of cancer here and not the gold medal, but I'm also aware that the former may seem just as unobtainable as the latter. Of course it does! Even with everything I've said so far you'll still be a long way from being ready to welcome cancer into your life as I did, but at least now it's a possibility. If it happened to me, it *can* happen to you. Why couldn't it?

Before you fill the space left by that question with any number of reasons why not, let me step in as your coach and get you back to your readiness training. I want to talk about buses and how to catch them. You may think that to catch a bus you simply need to know what time it goes and where from, but that's secondary to knowing:

    a)   that buses exist
    b)   that you want to catch one and
    c)   how to recognise one when it comes along.

Being ready takes organisation *and* awareness.
You have to know what it is you're looking for.

5

Have you experienced yourself as you truly are? Aside from your fears, insecurities and all traces of ego? As I walked out of the hospital the day the doctor told me I had cancer that was the experience I had. It wasn't what I expected, and I didn't see it coming, but I recognised it for what it was and I knew it was what I'd been waiting for.

The day started like any other—I had work to do and I was going to do it regardless of the circumstances! So off to the hospital I went with a bag full of research papers, some yellow post-its® and a pen. I was reviewing papers when called for my initial examination, and still trying to jam them into my bag as I walked into the consulting room. I was stressing about time as I waited for my ultrasound examination, worried whether I would finish all I had to do that day. And work was still on my mind as I waited for my results. Only with the diagnosis did it change. The clock started ticking. Thirty minutes, then nothing would be the same. Nothing of significance happened in those thirty minutes. Nothing was said to transform me. I had no enlightening thoughts. It was a transition time, that's all. I was already ready, but I needed time to adjust.

I remember following the breast-care nurse along the corridor after the diagnosis, straight ahead for thirty or so paces, a turn to the left, half as far again and a left into her office. I remember sitting in that office, both of us in front of her desk, me to the left and her to the right. I remember the way she talked to me, with an air of practised calm and reassurance, voice soft and gentle, body leaning forward slightly, heart reaching out. I remember standing to leave her office and turning to face the door.

What I don't remember is sound. I can't hear my feet in the corridor or doors opening or nurses' voices or humming machinery. Instead I hear an absence of sound, not as if sound has been muffled, but as if it has been taken away. And it's the same with feelings. I cannot access any feelings I had at that time, none at all. And when I try, all I get is a sense of something parting slowly in front of me, moving aside all that is there. This is not a parting of the Red Sea. There is no narrow channel that is always overshadowed and threatened by the weight of the water on each side. Instead it is a relaxed and gentle parting, as a mother would use when moving the edges of a blanket to lay her child inside.

6

But now I'm stuck and I don't know what to write next. It's a while since I wrote and I can't get back into the book. I stopped because some emotional issues were pushing so hard for my attention I had to deal with them; trying to write would have been pointless. These then fed through to some relationship issues I had to sort out. Then it was time to get ready for Christmas: cards to write; change of address cards to include (I'd moved six months before but told very few people); and presents to buy. Then I found a lump in my other breast.

That's interesting timing, isn't it? I find a second lump just as I'm telling you how cancer made me feel the first time round. At the time I knew it meant something—and I still feel that way—but I'm not going to understand it until I write it out. Maybe it happened simply to give me the next part of the book?

I found the first lump in bed. I felt a sharp pain in my breast, the left one, and put my hand there for comfort. I'd felt the pain before but never as sharply as then. Previously I'd believed it was my heart, not my breast, that was the source of the pain and that this stemmed from a broken heart! I'd been in love with a man for a couple of years—he didn't want a relationship with me—and I was completely stuck; nothing I tried got me out of it. So when I felt the pain of course it was my heart and of course it was to do with him. How could it be anything else? But when I put my hand there that time—at around 1am on 11th January 2001—there was a lump, just a small one, about the size of a pea.

Panic is the right word to describe my reaction: panic, fear and disbelief. When I felt the lump my hand shot away as if I'd chanced upon something hot and therefore dangerous to the touch. My breathing stopped and my limbs became rigid, allowing me to focus my senses on what was happening. Then fear struck—when everything stops, fear rushes in—and one word lunged into my head.

Cancer!

I lay frozen with fear. The only way out of that space was to put my hand there again, to the place that had caused the panic, to see if the lump was still there. It was. When I took my hand away and put it back again, the lump was there. If I moved to a different position, the lump remained. If I sat up then lay down again, the lump stayed the same. Nothing shifted it. No matter how much I wanted it *not* to be there, there it was. I'd gone to bed as me, now it was me and a lump.

I did what most people do in my situation, I phoned my doctor. But it was 1:30am and all the overnight service told me to do was to call again in the morning. It wasn't an emergency to them—but it was to me! It was a completely unexpected occurrence and a potentially highly dangerous one, and it demanded my full and immediate attention. And that's what the lump was about: getting my attention.

And the new lump has the same purpose—although this time it isn't cancer because it doesn't need to be. I no longer need cancer to help me sort my life out—but I do need a scare or two to keep me on track. You see I suffer from the terrible disease of complacency: complacency and the need to be liked. Both have done me far more damage than cancer ever did.

PART TWO

7

Because cancer looks like a villain, i.e. ugly, dark and dangerous, we assume it is one. Even now my parents tell of recently diagnosed cancer cases as they always have done—with hushed voices, with a knowledge of how terrible it is, and with a feeling of sadness for the sufferer and their family.

On one level I shouldn't be telling you this because it gives you room to say, "what use is she if she can't even get her parents to see things from her point of view!"

I take your point, but in my defence I'll say this: You, as yet, know nothing of my relationship with my parents, nor of their readiness or willingness to hear what I have to say. Some people get what I'm saying with relative ease, while others need a lot more words before they can begin to understand. Some people—most people—need a whole book.

If you see cancer as the villain then, by definition, you see yourself as the hero. Why? Because villain is defined (in Chambers English Dictionary[1]) as "a violent, malevolent or unscrupulous evil-doer...the wicked enemy of the hero or heroine in a story or play...".

I don't see cancer as a villain because I know that when it comes to me leading a full and fulfilling life, with me being the best that I can be, the biggest villain I have to face is myself. When I look back at my life I can see that any problems I've encountered are down to me—how *I* dealt with what life threw at me. Cancer is the hero of my piece because it stepped in and stopped me making a mess of my life. It showed me where I was going wrong and how to go forward.

As you probably don't see cancer in this way, it's time for me to turn attention away from me and towards you for a while. If that scares you, don't worry. Can anything I say be worse than having cancer? But if you're not scared, maybe you should be. Maybe you have much to lose from facing truth. And that, after all, is what cancer is about.

Truth and reality.
Reality and truth.

8

When you discovered your cancer, did you ask: "Why me?" Most people do. It's a common response. So common it's not even questioned. But this begs the further question: "Why not you?" Why, when one in three people get cancer[2], shouldn't you?

While I didn't ask 'why me?' after diagnosis I did think 'it can't be happening to me!' when I found the lump, however this phase was short lived. The day after I found the lump my general practitioner told me it probably wasn't cancer owing to: my age—mid thirties; my family history—no breast cancer in the family; that the lump hurt—most cancerous breast lumps do not cause pain; and the location of the lump itself—it wasn't in the place where cancers tend to occur. Then the lump grew very quickly—from a pea to a plum in a month—and lumps that grow that quickly tend to be cysts not cancer. So by the time I reached hospital the possibility that it was cancer had been pushed from my mind. It was a cyst: it had to be. Everybody said it was a cyst and 'things like cancer don't happen to me'. I'm mentioning this because 'it can't be happening to me!' and 'why me?' are manifestations of the same belief, i.e. that cancer happens to other people—not anyone in particular, just not me! We don't all hold this belief, but most of us do.

But what of the others? Those who do see cancer differently? Take, for example, women with breast cancer in the family, some of whom choose a voluntary bilateral mastectomy, i.e. removal of both breasts without an immediate medical need, so clear are they that cancer is a threat to them. While this may seem extreme, to these women—and I'm not being so bold as to speak on behalf of them here, I'm simply trying to explain their actions as best I can—this is the best solution. To help you understand this point of view let's talk about breast cancer for a while. Maybe you don't know much about it. Maybe you think it's a 'lesser' cancer—whatever that is. Maybe you think that after a breast is removed, all will be well. For those of you who don't know, and for those of you who are misinformed, here are the facts.

Breast cancer can kill. And kill it does to the tune of 13,000 women in the UK each year (about one third of the 40,000 cases diagnosed annually[3]) and 40,000 in the US (210,000 new cases annually[4]). Most breast cancer is invasive[5], which means that the cancer cells can live outside the breast and spread to other parts of the body. Breast cancer spreads by invading the lymphatic or blood vessels. These carry cancer cells to other parts of the body where they form other tumours called metastases. It's this that makes the disease more serious[6], i.e. it tends to be the secondary cancers that kill you.

The potential for a tumour to spread is measured in terms of 'grading'[7]. My cancer was grade III, which is the most aggressive form and explains why the lump grew so quickly. The prognosis for patients with grade III tumours is poor[8]. Following my mastectomy I was given only a 50% chance of surviving ten years. This increased after chemotherapy and again when I made it past the two-year mark (most recurrences are in the first two years after surgery). And I'll say while it's fresh in my mind, and when it may be a niggling doubt in yours, that, despite breast cancer being as dangerous for me as it was, I really do think of it as a hero.

But back to the focus of this part. I didn't have breast cancer in the family, I'd not been seriously ill before and, like many of us, I took my health for granted. So it didn't even cross my mind that cancer may happen to me. And, more importantly—certainly from the perspective of why I got cancer in the first place—I had, at one level, forgotten there was a 'me' at all. To explain what I mean by that I need to draw a distinction between a life in which you are the central driving force, and one where things happen to you and you deal with the consequences. Where I was before cancer was the second of these; where I am now is the first.

Before cancer I was a victim, and it's interesting to look up that word in the dictionary—"a living being offered as a sacrifice; one subjected to death, *suffering* or ill treatment: a prey: a *sufferer*"—because I didn't suffer with cancer, I did all of my suffering *before* I had cancer. I've told you something of my pre-cancer days—husband leaving, single mother, need to find work, unrequited love—but it's not so much what was happening as why that's important here.

Something happened a few minutes ago that will help me explain this. It's a very small incident that without explanation could be seen as both insignificant and irrelevant. But I *know* it's important—my body tells me so—and it's happened now, just when I need it. So it must be the way forward. A feeling in my body drew my attention to the incident I am about to describe. If you remember, the key to developing *knowing* is to listen to what your body wants and do it. Or to enlarge on that, to let your body guide by paying attention to the sensations, feelings and emotions it creates. Here's an example of this in action.

The feeling I have is in my chest, in my heart chakra[9].

The feeling didn't start in my chest though, rather it grew out of my body in the same way that a mist appears: seemingly out of nowhere, at first hardly detectable by the senses, but gradually increasing in intensity until it reaches the point where it has a discernible being. When I noticed the feeling it was at this early stage of formation. It was very subtle and something I could easily have dismissed or ignored if I was in that frame of mind, or too busy to give it space to grow. But, luckily, I acknowledged the feeling and turned my attention to it, and so my awareness of it developed alongside and at the same pace as the feeling itself.

The feeling was one of uneasiness and, as soon as I became aware of it, I knew it was linked to a recent 'phone call. Thinking about it now, the feeling must have started to form within my body as soon as I put the 'phone down. As I thought about the call, so the feeling grew. When fully formed throughout my body, mainly in the torso, it concentrated itself to my heart chakra in the way that a genie returns to a bottle: condensing its being into a focused stream of vapour that aims at then fills the target void. And it was here in my heart chakra that the feeling peaked in intensity, causing a tightening of my chest and inducing a sensation of pain.

I didn't have to think long about the call to know what the issue was. I'd allowed the person on the other end of the 'phone to stop me doing as I intended. How did that happen? I picked up signals that she was not happy and, in direct response to these and without thinking about it, changed my request to meet her wants/needs and not my own. Here's how I remember the conversation. I speak first.

"Are you the person I spoke to earlier?"

"No, that must have been Mrs Brown."

"Can I speak to her?"

"I'll see if I can find her."

"No, don't worry. Can you take a message instead?..."

It's not obvious from that what happened, is it? And I guess that's the point. These things are very subtle and control us without us realising it. It's not what was said but how it was said that made the difference. My actions were determined by the woman's tone of voice.

There was almost a sigh when she said, "No, that must have been Mrs Brown", which suggested she was already anticipating what I was going to say in a negative way. Indeed, the line was spoken as if by an actor asked to convey both an expectation that Mrs Brown had promised the earth, and an anticipation that she (and not Mrs Brown) would be called upon to deliver that promise. "I'll see if I can find her" was similarly weighted, this time with slight annoyance. When she'd finished I could almost hear, "but I haven't really got time for this and I've no idea where she will be!" And so, because of how this person spoke to me and without really thinking about it, I changed my request from "can I speak to her?" which is what I wanted to do, to "can you take a message...?"

"So what!" You may be thinking. "Does this really matter?" The answer is yes. One thousand times yes. For it is in such conversations that we give ourselves away. When we allow ourselves to be diverted from our purpose—from speaking our truth—we lose a part of ourselves, and if we do this enough times, with enough people and in enough circumstances, in the end there is not enough of us left to sustain who we are.

Our bodies try to stop this process by drawing attention

to these incidents—remember this started with me describing a feeling that grew out of my body—but how many of us pay attention to such messages? How many of us are even aware of them or are guilty of blocking them? And because we don't pay attention to our bodies when they speak to us nicely, they eventually give up the polite talk and call in the big boys, i.e. cancer or some other major illness. By the time cancer steps in you are well past polite conversation.

Cancer does not talk, it screams.
And what does it scream?
You! You! You! You! You! You! You!

We started with the question, 'Why me?' The answer is because there *is* a you. And it is because you have forgotten who that person is that cancer comes. A hero whose sole purpose is your salvation.

9

This is heavy, isn't it? I feel the need for some light relief. Or maybe that's me pandering to what I think you want to hear or can handle reading. It's something a friend of mine worries about when it comes to this book—she's concerned you'll get the message that cancer is your fault. I can see where she's coming from. What I'm saying does imply that you have cancer because of the choices you've made and the path you've taken. My friend sees this as a bad thing— as may you—but I don't. Cancer is not a punishment. This is not about blame. Our points of view differ because we see cancer differently. How we feel about cancer, how we relate to it and how we deal with it, depends on what we believe it to be. I believe cancer can be an incredibly powerful positive force. Most people, because cancer can kill, see it only as a bad thing.

I need to check your relationship to what I'm saying. Although I can't allow myself to dilute what I have to say in response to any noises you may be making, I must have these in mind when deciding on my approach. I know what I have to say may not be easy for you to hear. And as a communicator and your teacher, I have a responsibility to account for that as best I can, while at the same time not allowing myself to be pushed from my path or persuaded from speaking my truth.

I wondered what you thought when I wrote the word 'teacher'. I doubt anyone could object to the word 'communicator' but the word 'teacher', that could get some people's backs up. Maybe you're one of them? Maybe you don't think you need a teacher or think I'm being impudent in calling myself one? Maybe use of the word has annoyed you so much you want to stop reading the book!

Looking at the dictionary definition of the word teacher—and what better source have we when it comes to the meaning of words?—you have no reason to be angry with me, because according to this definition I'm not over-stepping the mark. A teacher is "one whose profession is, or whose talent is the ability to impart knowledge, practical skill or understanding." It's OK for me to use the word teacher because reading this book can give you a better understanding of yourself, what it means to be a person with cancer and some practical skills to help you along the way. And knowledge? That's what this book is about—helping you to develop your *knowing* so that you can guide yourself through life and continually improve and develop your relationship with yourself. Therefore, if you have a problem with the word teacher, although you may feel angry and annoyed with me, it's you who has the problem. And I need to draw your attention to it, for if I don't, I'll lose you.

When you read this book (or talk to other people) you do so in the context of what you believe about the world. Therefore, what you believe about the world influences what you feel about this book (or that conversation). The discussion of the word teacher should have, if you weren't aware of it already, opened your eyes to this. It's the same with cancer. Not many people hear the word cancer in a purely medical sense, i.e. "a carcinoma or disorderly growth of epithelial cells which invade adjacent tissue and spread by the lymphatics and blood vessels to other parts of the body" (Chambers). Instead, the word is heard in the context of what society believes it to be, as revealed by the manner in which the word is used as a figure of speech, and figuratively (as defined in the dictionary) cancer is "any corroding evil"! Given this, is it any surprise that we react to a diagnosis of cancer in the way that we do?

Your belief systems influence this book and in particular the way it's written. I could tell you everything about cancer and my philosophy in a couple of chapters, maybe less if I was very economical with words, but if I did that this book wouldn't work. What I have to say is *so* different from the conventional view of cancer that if I just came out and said it, it would be too easy for you to dismiss or ignore. This has happened to me many times in my everyday life. People discover I had cancer and are interested to know more, often because they're surprised it happened to me, someone relatively young and healthy looking. However, when I start to speak about my experience, nineteen times out of twenty the conversation is one-sided and doesn't last long. I start to say how it was for me and the other person doesn't know what to say or how to react and the conversation ends.

What I have to say is so different that most people cannot cope with it. Therefore, it cannot be said quickly or directly and I have to come at you from the side.

You know too much
About the way things are
To be told anything different.
Your world is flat
While mine is round.
And the last thing you want
Is for me to reveal that to you.

And so I have to draw on the wisdom of my body in writing this book. I have to allow it, through the creative process, to lead. Therefore I'm going to talk to you about my hair. Yes, *really*.

10

I had a haircut last week and I hate it. Everyday I get up, look in the mirror and get angry and/or upset about my hair. What do I hate about it? Everything. It's everything I didn't want in a haircut and yet it's what I ended up with. Worst of all, this is my fault. The hairdresser did as I asked. When I go to the hairdressers I have a problem saying: "this is what I want". Because of this my haircuts have developed a pattern. 1) I have a haircut I don't like. 2) It grows out, I get used to styling it and I start to like it. 3) My hair starts to get too long but I put off going to the hairdressers. 4) My hair gets so long it's a mess and I have to have it cut, but by this time I don't care what the hairdresser does as anything will be better than what I've got. 5) I have a haircut I don't like.

Last week in an attempt to break the pattern I bought a hair magazine, highlighted the styles I liked and took it with me to the hairdressers. Why then did I end up with a haircut I didn't like? Because I dare not get the magazine out of my bag! Instead I mumbled a few words that ended with, "cut it the same as last time," i.e. the same as the last haircut I didn't like. I know it's ridiculous but at the time it was all I could do. My fears and insecurities got the better of me and I couldn't act differently. What was I most afraid of? The hairdresser's reaction when I showed him a picture of how I wanted to look. I was afraid he'd raise his eyebrows in a 'you can't be serious!' manner or that he'd laugh at the ridiculousness of me believing I could look that way.

At the time I didn't know these were my fears. Looking at myself in the hairdresser's mirror I was afraid—afraid that I'd end up with a haircut I didn't like—but the real fears that were driving my actions were hidden. That's how fear works, isn't it? Rarely does it sit out in the open where it can be seen, understood and tackled head on. Instead it hides in the shadows, just out of sight, menacing you with its presence. It makes you believe it is bigger than it is, that it cannot be conquered, and that the last thing you should do is to look it in the face.

My fear (of being considered a fool) controlled me because I didn't stop to look at it and take time to work out what it was. I allowed it to be a nebulous, all-powerful presence and so that is what it was. And because of that, I ended up with a bad haircut. My bad haircut is a physical manifestation of fear. I allowed fear to lead me and ended up with exactly what I didn't want and am suffering because of it. Fear *always* works this way. It tricks us into following the wrong path—to walk in the dark instead of the light—and it needs us to do this so that it can survive. Fear cannot exist without us to feed it. If we do not give it our energy, it ceases to be. That's not an easy thing for any of us to do but that's where cancer comes in. You can use cancer to stop being afraid.

What is cancer there for, if not to be used?
And what better way to use it than to conquer fear?

Your body gave you cancer for a multitude of reasons but two main ones stand out. It wants you to pay attention to you—the true you that lays long forgotten—and it wants you to use cancer to get closer to this person. Think of it as a shovel or a lever that can help move aside all the stuff that stands in the way of being the true you.

In case some of you are struggling with this—maybe you find the idea of using cancer abhorrent or amoral—you need to know you don't have a choice about this. Cancer *will* bring you closer to the true you: either you use cancer to get closer to your true self by facing the fears and the issues it raises, or your body allows cancer to take over, to kill you and reunite you with your true self that way.

Does this sound shocking and too much to take in? Some things always will the first time they're said. To make it easier, I'll talk about God. Don't worry, you don't need to believe in God for this book to be all that it can for you, but it is to God that I need to go next.

I I

Why do I believe in God? Because I have experienced God. It's as simple as that. The difficulty comes in describing what I've experienced and in explaining why God is the best name for it. I'll start by saying that my belief in God is a new thing. When I mentioned God to my mum she was shocked. Thirteen years ago I'd very much not believed in God, so much so that a church wedding was out of the question. It wasn't that I was anti-God—I opted for a registry office so as not to be hypocritical—but that I had no experience of God on which to base a belief. This changed when I got cancer, not because I was afraid of death and needed something to believe in, but because I began to have experiences that I am now calling God.

I didn't want to believe in God, I wasn't looking for God, and for a long time I struggled with my path. I particularly worried about the place of God in my life and in this book. God is a hugely controversial term and just mention of the word is enough to enrage some people and turn off many others. Because of this I've looked for another word to use but, try as I might, I can't find one. God is the only word that's big enough to encompass the length and breadth of my experiences, their depth and intensity, and their magic and wonder.

In my experience God is an energy: a universal, positive energy that is both eternal and infinite. This energy is important to me and out of my experience of it my philosophy has grown. The energy I am calling God surrounds us at all times and when we're being our true selves we tap into it. The energy is here to support and to guide us and our souls are part of it—'the little bit of God in all of us'.

Our bodies separate us from this energy and connect us to it. Without our bodies we are one with this energy, i.e. when we die we return to God. Through our bodies we get to experience what it means to be alive, i.e. to be separate from God, but if we are open we get to experience God too. It's this experience that keeps me going and gives my life purpose. By moving closer to my true self, I move closer to this thing I call God and the payback is how that makes me feel. The feelings that arise from contact with God energy are without equal.

If you don't believe in God, don't worry. This book can still be for you. Why? Because your body determines whether you live or die. That's not difficult to grasp, most of us realise we're reliant on our bodies for life, but what we fail to grasp is the real nature of this relationship and especially our body's role in it. Think of your body as a separate entity—a separate person if you like.

Inside my head I said "hello Lesley" to my body and my eyes filled with tears. Without probing deeper I don't know what these mean, but I know for me tears are a sign of emotional truth and thus the right way to go. Repeating the phrase, 'hello Lesley', the tears come again and are accompanied by a feeling in my torso—in that place between my belly button and my heart—and a fear around my shoulders. Being me, I allow fear to dominate and start to edit this section rather than going deeper to find out what underlies the feeling. I'm no different from you, you see. I'm still driven by fear and insecurity, but maybe a little better at realising this and switching across to a different path.

Time has passed since I wrote the last paragraph and the emotions that were driving the tears have long since passed. I tried to do the 'hello Lesley' exercise again but what came was not the same as before. My next thought was to scrap the section and start again but that would not be the right thing to do, not in this instance. This has something to do with the way life is — I caught a glimpse of a truth when I considered scrapping the paragraph but it was fleeting and now is gone.

That's how it is with *knowing* — that's bodily knowing and not the know-it-all type — sometimes it arrives complete as a sudden realisation or fundamental truth, but more often than not it creeps up on you. You catch a glimpse of it out of the corner of your eye. It flits into your thoughts. It hides in the words of others. And it continues to show itself until you are ready, or rather able, to see it in its entirety.

Each time the knowing shows itself, how much we are able to grasp depends not on the knowing but on ourselves and in particular on the space we give it. We are like a camera that has its shutter firmly closed. When the shutter does open it does so for just a fraction of a second, which is not long, but long enough to let in the light.

12

The knowing I caught a glimpse of is linked with the past. Our lives are a series of steps, each one following the next. Sometimes we walk in a straight line but more often we meander, so much so that it can take one thousand steps to get somewhere instead of just the one. Me greeting my body and listening to the response was one step. Other things that happened between that time and me picking up the threads of the book (over the course of a few days) were also steps. Other things were me treading water. How do you know the difference between a step and staying still? Oh, you know, but probably your shutter remains firmly closed on this one. It's one of those cases where you already know but refuse to see it.

There's a widely accepted belief that as we get older time moves more quickly, with years rushing by as quickly as months passed when we were younger. This is not my experience of life. It was. But it's not now.

If time appears to pass more quickly it's because you're no longer taking steps forward; you're simply treading water. This isn't easy to understand if you've not seen it for yourself because it seems to counter other experiences when it comes to time. But that's how you fool yourself for in reality there is no difference at all. If you're waiting for an appointment with nothing to do, time passes slowly; yet if you're busy, time can fly by. When it comes to taking steps forward in life—emotional and spiritual steps, that is—we fill in non-busy times with distractions. Thus we believe we're taking steps when we're not. Indeed some people's lives become so focused on creating distractions that's all they do.

The way you measure time was set during childhood. Remember as a small child a day seemed to last forever and a week was so long as to be incomprehensible? This is because of the speed of change. To a young child everything is changing and nothing remains the same; every day there are new skills to acquire and things to explore. A day is experienced in terms of these changes and the pace of the internal clock set: one day equals ten changes, for example. As you get older and the speed of change slows, you may experience ten changes not once a day but once a week or once a month, and if you are very stuck a whole year or more may pass with little or no change.

As a result of having cancer—or rather, as a result of experiencing life with the benefit of cancer—I realised that I love things to move quickly, i.e. for my life to be full of changes. And how ironic that was! Because before cancer my life hardly changed at all. What do I mean by changes? For me these are mainly emotional—often a release of trapped emotion leading to a new level of awareness, or a facing up to reality leading to a greater degree of clarity and peace.

Because my life has changed since cancer, time now moves more quickly and more slowly than it has ever done. Some days I have so many emotional shifts and realisations that when looking back, that very morning seems as if it were days ago. And time moving slowly? That comes out of the fullness of life. Life being so full of exploration and growth that time almost stops, for it is no longer relevant. To help you understand this, and me and why cancer was such a gift, I need to go back to the bad old days before cancer. To that phase in my life when I moved inexorably slowly and time seemed to bind my hands and feet.

As I turn my attention to that time tears come to my eyes and I am filled with sadness. This was a bleak and desolate time, a time of misery, and it's this I was rescued from. I was off track and relentlessly pushing in the direction of a dead end and although I was miserable and so there was a clue for me there, I had no idea how far from my path I was. And, having cancer, it must be the same for you. Although maybe you're so good at distracting yourself and at make-believe you don't realise you need saving. Or, so set in your ways and so sure of yourself that you think life was great until you got cancer. How so, so wrong you can be.

13

It's the difference between real and imagined steps that's important here. That, and getting you to see and accept the difference. Why? Because when you're treading water you believe you're taking great strides forward. That's the catch—and a big one too.

I've been distracted by the window cleaner and, as I allow life as well as my body to direct me, I'm going to share with you our conversation. I'd just finished the first paragraph when the doorbell rang. As my office is upstairs it took a while to get to the front door especially as, in my hurry to get up, I knocked over a plate and a cup on the way. By the time I got downstairs the window cleaner was knocking. In the time it took to unlock the door and remove the chain we started calling to each other. I shouted, "Wait a minute!" in what was for me a surprisingly grumpy way.

He shouted, "Sorry!"

And I, while unlocking the door and removing the chain, shouted, "No worries, I shouldn't be so grumpy!"

Blah, blah, blah! I hate reporting in that way because I find it extremely tedious. The point of the story is that when I opened the door I thought the window cleaner called me an "impatient git", when in reality he said it about himself. How do I know this? Because believing I'd been insulted I took offence. Thus when he asked whether I wanted my windows cleaned I, not surprisingly, said no. However, as he started to walk away I told him why I'd said no and we worked it out. Consequently, having discovered the truth, on shutting the door I realised that what I wanted *was* to have my windows cleaned—I've been in this house over eight months and have cleaned only one window once (!)—so I went outside and called him back. He's cleaning the windows as I type. Oh! How I love a happy ending.

But to the point of the story and why this is important now: breaking free of the illusory world and stepping forward into reality. It's only possible to tread water and at the same time believe you're taking great strides forward if you're out of touch with reality. This is so, so important and anything you can do to break down the walls of illusion is good. One way is to share your illusions with others. If I'd not told the window cleaner I was annoyed with him for calling me a git, I'd not have discovered my misunderstanding. And instead of sitting here with clean windows and a happy heart—he's a nice guy and we had a chat when he'd finished—I'd be sitting here annoyed at the impudence of some people and with dirty windows to boot!

Even though this appears to be a trivial example, it's not. Well, it is and it isn't. Trivial is not only "of little importance" but also "to be found anywhere", and that's the point. Everyday we have many interactions of the type I've described. That's many opportunities to say things as they are for you and to test whether you're living in reality. You can change your life overnight simply by being straight with people, at all times and in all circumstances. I'm not there yet, but it is my goal. And, of course, I was the very opposite of this before I had cancer.

14

My childhood was the opposite of my son's. Of course it was. Isn't that what we parents do? Put most of our energies into making sure our children don't have to endure what we had to endure? My son is going to grow up not wanting to talk about his feelings because I put so much emphasis on this (if he's to rebel, that is). While with me it wasn't so much a case of not wanting to talk, as not knowing that I wanted to talk nor how to do so. Indeed I still act this way sometimes. In fact it happened just a couple of weeks ago. I'm reticent about discussing this though—the feeling I have is a mixture of boredom and anger—but because it's appeared I'm going to explore it. If an emotion is present it's your body talking to you, so it's best to look at it and not put it to one side.

When I focus on the anger I can feel it in my chest (in my heart chakra) and my jaw tightens as if I'm preparing to bite someone—not that this is a habit of mine! Focusing on my jaw and teeth it feels as if the anger has moved from my body into my mouth and I am ready to spit it at someone—not that I make a habit of that either! Sitting with it for a bit longer the anger diffuses slightly, my eyes narrow and all of my attention focuses on waiting—waiting for someone to strike. Everything points to me being in defensive mode in readiness for a fight. This bodily reaction has been triggered by the memory I'm about to share with you. With its reaction my body is talking to me and showing me the way; preparing me for the steps I need to take and showing me what they should be.

Five weeks ago I saw a nutritionist. I didn't want to change my diet—it's hard, isn't it?—but at Christmas when I found the lump in my other breast and had some other physical problems I finally took the advice of my acupuncturist and booked an appointment. To my breast-care specialists the second lump was "lumpy tissue and a few cysts", i.e. nothing to worry about, but from the perspective of traditional Chinese medicine the diagnosis is different. Change in the breast is not a good thing and for me is considered one step back along the road to cancer. And however much I like the way I am when I have cancer, it's far too dangerous a route to freedom for me to choose. So off to the nutritionist I went.

The regime she prescribed is strict and a long way from the diet of most Westerners. Even for a vegetarian, organic-food eating, alcohol-, black tea- and coffee-free person such as me big changes have been required. To reduce the load on my liver, to level out my blood sugar and to have a diet that's just right for me, it's no wheat, no dairy, no potatoes, no corn, no rice and no sugar. All nuts are to be soaked for 12 hours before eating, pulses soaked for 24 and 'rested' for another day to sprout before cooking. Sounds a nightmare? It's not. But I have had a few problems that I'll come to in a minute. In fact as soon as I started the diet I began to feel the benefits, and looking at it realistically it was the only way for me to go. Like giving up alcohol it's the right time and I'm ready to do it. And as that's a story that almost always makes people sit up and listen, I'll tell it now.

I haven't had an alcoholic drink for over 10 months, which for most people is astonishing to hear; especially when I add that I never want to drink again. Alcohol is such an integral part of our culture and the only widely accepted (and legal) way of relaxing, that to most people it's inconceivable I would want to give it up. Particularly as I didn't drink a lot and certainly didn't have a problem with it, nor was it something I'd considered or even wanted to do. Why give it up then? My standard line is, "my body and life conspired to make it happen", and I guess that's what gets people's attention. That and the fact they are surprised anyone could be alcohol-free, let alone enjoy it.

I knew something was afoot. I had a busy weekend arranged, out on Friday and on Saturday, when I received an invitation for the Thursday evening. Normally I would have refused, for babysitting reasons mainly, not thinking it fair on my son to be away from home three nights in a row, but on this occasion I wanted to go — I was certain of it — and that's what got my attention. I *knew* something was going to happen. Of course, being me, I thought I'd meet a gorgeous man — no such luck! — and as it turned out it was, at the time, something completely unexpected.

Thursday evening I felt unwell and although I wanted to go out I knew if I drank alcohol I'd not survive the night let alone make it through the weekend. So I decided to drink water. It wasn't the first time I'd been out without alcohol but it was the first time I'd gone from pub to club, including a dance, completely sober. It wasn't a bad experience or especially a good one; I had a fairly reasonable time and didn't feel too uncomfortable on the dance floor. My perspective changed, however, in the morning.

When I woke I felt good, much better than after a normal night on the town, and when I looked in the mirror I was amazed. Not drinking made *such* a difference to how I looked. Not that I normally drank lots, say five single vodkas with cranberry — that was my signature drink. Now it's sparkling mineral water, no ice or lemon.

It was partly an age thing but mainly a question of hydration. I stopped drinking at 38 and a few months, an age when one's skin is not quite as youthful and elastic as it once was. Although to go back, or rather forward, to the new diet, my skin looks better now than it ever has. But that aside, the older you are the less resilient your body is (skin, liver, and everything else) to the effects of alcohol—and that's why the impact of not drinking was so noticeable. Instead of dehydrating my body with alcohol, I'd hydrated it with mineral water and looked fabulous as a result. That's what I saw the next day and it was enough to make me give non-drinking another go. And that's where life was so generous—or clever, depending how you look at it—because it gave me the opportunity to do so that very day *and* the day after in two completely different settings. It was the experience of those two evenings that got me hooked.

Friday was a re-run of the night before. However, whereas I'd been a martyr on Thursday for not being able to drink, this time it was a game: 'will I be able to do it again and maybe even enjoy it this time?' My experience on the dance-floor clinched it. It was as if a bit of me had been freed. I was willing to make a fool of myself and I was more carefree. And to a person who has spent most of her adult life being uptight, and who is still prone to bouts of seriousness, that was very, very welcome. Spurred on by success I didn't drink on Saturday either, this time at a house party; something I normally hated and would not have agreed to go to had it not been the party of a very dear friend. Not only was the party OK for me without alcohol, I enjoyed it. I was open to talk to people rather than being afraid of what I might say or what they might think, which is something that held me back for years. And the outcome of this, and the realisation that keeps me alcohol-free, is an awareness that alcohol doesn't do it for me anymore. No longer does it free me from my insecurities and hang-ups as it did in the beginning; instead it seems to inhibit me in some way.

As soon as life and my body conspired to make me give up alcohol it was clear I shouldn't be drinking. Alcohol takes you away from yourself and as my goal is to get closer to the real me it doesn't make sense for me to drink; it's one step away from where I want to be and that's one step too far. But I wouldn't have seen this on my own. Because drinking is such a part of the 'enjoying yourself' culture, without a little help I'd have been unable to even contemplate giving it up.

And that's why my body—and yours—is so wonderful. Because it always—and I mean *always*—knows best.

But back to the present and the new diet. This is another case of my body taking me somewhere that a) I didn't want to go but that b) is absolutely where I need to go, given who I am and what I'm committed to.

Even though my diet is paying dividends in some areas—my pulses[10] are already stronger than they've been for some time and remember the glowing skin!—it's still not working in terms of my digestion. The issue in itself isn't a problem, but how I'm handling it is. I'm OK now but go back a couple of weeks and this wasn't the case at all. I knew things weren't as they should be but didn't realise how much this was getting me down. Only when I talked to a friend did it come out. I started crying and saying how awful it was and how hard it had been.

The key to letting out the emotion was feeling safe. Because my friend had seen the same nutritionist and had also followed a restrictive diet, I knew she wouldn't try to persuade me away from mine or try to influence me in any way. I say "knew", but I only realised this later. Before I let the emotion out, I had no idea it was in there. Why is that? It's a way of being I developed when very small in order to survive in an unsupportive environment. Instead of letting out emotion and making myself vulnerable to others, I learned to suppress it to the point that it disappeared from view—that's mine as well as everyone else's! And having brought that up it really is time to go back to the beginning—life before cancer: my childhood.

PART THREE

15

I'll start with me falling in the river. Why? Because it popped into my head and therefore it must be the perfect place to start. I was about three when it happened and thinking of that time brings tears to my eyes. There is no memory associated with these tears, save for the trigger, and no emotion associated with them either. Thinking about them, or rather focusing on them, they seem to be about loss.

Saying to myself, "falling in the river", there is a sensation in my torso, in the solar plexus—a feeling of yearning which again leads to tears. Something is trapped here, I can see it in the cycle: tears, yearning, tears, yearning, tears, yearning, tears. What am I yearning for? A lost childhood. The answer signalled by a rush of emotion from belly to throat.

We were walking by the river close to where I was brought up. That's my mum, my nanny (my paternal grandmother), my sister (must have been a babe in arms) and me. Yellow is the predominant colour—the hot, white yellow of the summer sun and the pale, lemon yellow of my hand-knitted cardigan. The tears (that have come again) stem from me gaining access to my state of being at that time, the contrast between that and how I am now, and the time that has passed between. Thirty-six years of being less than.

I don't know what made me fall. Maybe I looked at my reflection in the water and leant too far. Maybe I caught sight of a fish and in my excitement slipped. But what made me fall is not important because the falling itself is significant here: significant for what it was and what it was not. I fell at the place where the boats moored, at the point where the river was deepest, and weighted down by my cardigan must have sank quickly to the bottom—but that is not my memory of falling. Instead I moved through the water as a leaf falls in autumn when there is no wind to influence its descent, not straight down but with a gentle swaying that both slows and eases the fall.

The tears have come again at the memory of this fall and in anticipation of the world into which I fell. They draw me forward. Stopping when I try to uncover their meaning but starting up again when I try to figure out why I am so lost without them. Finally they put me down in the place I need to be, in that watery green-hued world with the sounds of everyday life muffled from me. Where I feel—and this is what I've been building to—safe.

Safety is not what I felt at the time. Then it was wide-eyed wonder at the sights, sounds and feelings of a completely new experience. But stepping back into it now, safety is all I feel: safety and that underlying feeling of loss. But the loss is, I see now, just a way of avoiding the feeling of safety. It is one step away from the truth and thus one step away from the pain.

It would be easy for me to try to 'figure out' this issue of safety—figuring things out is my default response to everything—but that will not get me where I need to go. The truth will only emerge from my body and will not be given by my head. So I need to sit with the word "safety", and the backdrop of my watery world, and let the emotions flow. The answers *will* be given, if they are given space to be.

The memories our bodies retain for us hold the answers to the riddles of our lives. To uncover their secrets, look with your body and not with your mind. Feel your way to the truth, learning to use emotion and sensation as you have been taught to use reason and intellect. This is akin to meditation in that you allow the thoughts to come but don't hold onto them, waiting for a fuller picture to emerge. It's not an easy process but it is a fruitful one.

What makes it difficult? It's not easy to sit with emotion and let it lead. It's scary, it's unpredictable, and it hurts. And more than that, we're used to being in control — sometimes like a lion tamer with his whip, sometimes like a teacher with an unruly class of children, but always with the same aim: to keep order and ensure self-preservation. But what we fail to see with this approach is that in taming the lion we are, in reality, taming ourselves. And while this can never be the path to true and lasting happiness, we fool ourselves that it is.

I've been struggling with what to write next, and finally it's dawned on me that this may be because I'm afraid of what will be uncovered when I sit with the word "safety". Yes me, whose whole raison d'être is to get closer to the true me, is afraid of doing just that. There's that aspect to it (and I shall return to this later), but maybe I'm also not yet ready to go forward with this book. Although self-discovery and writing sometimes go hand-in-hand, at other times the writing has to wait. It's hard for me to see when it is such a time though. Because I want to finish the book I allow this want, unconsciously, to override the messages I get from my body, i.e. that when I sit with the word "safety" I cry and cry and cry.

And this ploughing on regardless gets me nowhere, other than to open the door to my fears and insecurities:

"I'll never finish this book. I've lost my thread and I'll never find it. I've headed off in the wrong direction. Who am I kidding when I think I can write a book?" So I'll let the tears come—all of them—and come back to you when I'm ready. Because until then there's no point continuing.

16

It's a day later and still the tears have not yet come. Sometimes life gets in the way of moving forward—I had to pick up my son from school and spend 'us' time together, then I was too tired and in a different space—and sometimes we need to take a break from the task—I spent this morning with a friend, drinking green tea and getting back to the place where I believe in myself again. Having brought myself here, I feel I can write about safety and allow this process to be the means of discovery. Whereas yesterday I was not strong enough for this approach, today it is OK. And this is part of what I'm trying to communicate and understand for myself: there are days when you can and days when you can't.

Some days are perfect for moving forward, while others are for recouping energy and taking time out simply to be. Distinguishing one from another is not easy, however. I always feel I should be writing whether I'm up to the task or not. I came back from spending time with my friend and felt alive and energised—back to the old me. Yet after only a few minutes at my keyboard trying to write this book, I again feel doubtful about myself and my abilities. I allowed my energy and enthusiasm to mask the fact that I still need to deal with the safety issue. I still need to cry.

Why do this? Because taking the short cut is easier. It's less painful and it gives me what I want, i.e. to write this book. Despite everything I stand for I'm prepared to do anything other than face up to the next truth. And because this is where we *all* fall down, I've written this book. If there's one thing to show you there's no such thing as a short cut and that facing up to reality is the only way forward, it's cancer. Once you've got it, there really is only the long haul.

And because I've brought that up, now would be a good time to look at what the long haul involves. This is not me avoiding the safety issue as you might think but me working up to it. Through my writing I'll get to a point where I'm able to face the truth—whatever it is. And—this is the magic of writing—I'll be tying the safety issue into what I'm about to say. Not that I have any idea how this will work, only a feeling that this will be the result.

17

It's two days later and I'm filled with fear. I've reached the place where, in order to go forward, I must face the issues I've been avoiding and that have, therefore, been holding me back. There's the personal issue — safety — and now, in order to get there, I've to deal with the aspect of cancer I'm most afraid of: the possibility of, or perhaps the inevitability of, your death.

I put the phrase "...or perhaps the inevitability of..." into the sentence after the rest was written and therein lies the heart of the problem, but also magically the way forward. Three years on from my cancer I'm still here, but for some of you this may not be the outcome, and what I've been afraid of — the fear has passed now that I've faced it head on — is how I'm going to talk to you about death. And the magical part of that sentence? The bringing into my consciousness an awareness of the inevitability of everyone's death, and a knowing that through a discussion of this I'll find a way forward.

The obvious thing about cancer is death. If there's one thing cancer does it's to bring the issue of mortality out of the background and into the foreground, albeit with the subtlety of a jumbo jet revving its engines outside your front door. The real issue, however, is that you'd not thought about it before. If you'd thought about and come to terms with your own death, that aspect of a cancer diagnosis wouldn't be such an issue, would it?

But thinking about death is not something we Westerners do. Our culture encourages the very opposite of an examination of mortality. We live in a world where the important things are, in terms of this discussion, looking young for as long as possible and saving for and enjoying a long retirement. There's an implicit assumption that we'll be around until, at the very least, our seventies, and that when we get there we'll look as if we're in our fifties—and shame on us if we don't!

So let's not look at what society tells us to see and believe, instead let's look at the facts, i.e. death rate statistics. Through these you'll see how you fit into the big picture and get a reality check on your views.

Likelihood of death per annum in England and Wales			
Age	Odds	Male	Female
Under 1	1 in	169	222
1 to 4	1 in	4000	5000
5 to 9	1 in	8333	10000
10 to 14	1 in	6250	9091
15 to 19	1 in	2041	4167
20 to 24	1 in	1282	3704
25 to 34	1 in	1064	2273
35 to 44	1 in	633	1064
45 to 54	1 in	256	400
55 to 64	1 in	103	167
65 to 74	1 in	37	59
75 to 84	1 in	14	20
85 and over	1 in	5	6

Data for 2002 from Table 6.1 *Deaths: Age and Sex, Numbers and Rates, 1976 onwards (England and Wales)*, Health Statistics Quarterly 21.

Women and men are considered separately because the rates are quite different. (Sorry guys, being male makes you more likely to die in any given year than us gals, save for babies under the age of 1.)

To explain the data I'll use myself, a 39-year-old woman, as an example. The odds of any woman in this age group dying this year are 1 in 1,064, i.e. for every 1,064 of us out there, one will die. The older you get, unsurprisingly, the chances of dying increase. By the time a woman reaches 45 her odds of dying are 1 in 400, and if she reaches 75 reduce to 1 in 20. The statistics assume that everyone in an age group is equally healthy and has an equal chance of dying. This is not the case—remember at one point my doctors gave me only a 50% chance of surviving ten years—but despite this, the data are a good starting point. They set out where you were before you had cancer and that place and your awareness of it is important.

To help you see what I see, think about winning the lottery. Though some of you will have no experience of it having never bought a ticket, I think (based on no data whatsoever) that you will be in the minority. Most people buy a ticket at least occasionally with some buying a number religiously each week. And it's to this last group that I'm particularly talking, although I think what I have to say will be of interest to everybody.

When asked what her ambition was a contestant on a gameshow said, "to win the lottery!" To that woman and others like her I'll say this: "You're more likely to wind up dead". The facts: at the age of 30 a woman is 118 times more likely to die than win the lottery this year, assuming she buys one ticket a week. She can up the odds of winning by purchasing more tickets but she needs to buy 119 tickets *per week every week for a year*, at a cost of £6,188, to make it more likely that she wins the jackpot than dies[11]. If she wants her partner to share her winnings (he was with her on the gameshow) she needs to buy 372 tickets every week for a year, at a cost of £19,344, to ensure that the odds of winning are greater than the odds of her or her partner dying[12].

If you want to know how many lottery tickets you need to buy every week for a year to make it more likely that you'll win the lottery than die, look at the table below.

Number of lottery tickets to be purchased *EACH WEEK* for the likelihood of winning the jackpot to exceed the likelihood of death in any one year				
	Male		Female	
Age	Tickets per week	Cost per annum	Tickets per week	Cost per annum
16 to 19	132	£6,864	65	£3,380
20 to 24	210	£10,920	73	£3,796
25 to 34	253	£13,156	119	£6,188
35 to 44	425	£22,100	253	£13,156
45 to 54	1,051	£54,652	673	£34,996
55 to 64	2,611	£135,772	1,611	£83,772
65 to 74	7,269	£377,988	4,558	£237,016
75 to 84	19,209	£998,868	13,446	£699,192
85 and over	53,784	£2,796,768	44,820	£2,330,640
Data for the UK lottery (you must be 16 or over to play or claim a prize). See notes 11 and 12 for information on how these data were calculated.				

The problem is not that the woman plays the lottery but that it is her ambition to win. An ambition should be realistic and attainable, for if it is not, you end up disillusioned and disappointed or living in a dream world.

It is in this last place that most of us in the Western world live. The proof? You believe you might win the lottery—odds of nearly 14 million-to-one—but it comes as a shock that you might get cancer—odds of 1 in 3 per lifetime—or that you might die. I'm sorry, but that's delusional. Look at the facts.

> The only thing guaranteed in this life, is death.
> Ain't no way round it, that's the truth.

How is it that we fail to see the truth? Because it's more comfortable that way. Consider two days: one spent planning how you'll spend your lottery winnings, the other considering your death. Which is more attractive? The first one, of course! Even I feel that way and I know where I'm going with this. There's something that pulls us towards the first and keeps us well and truly away from the second. We like to think of nice things, to see ourselves in good situations and with the time and wherewithal to do as we please. We don't like to see ourselves going through bad times, at the end of the line and with no control over our destiny. But it's as a result of facing up to death that I have a life that I want and enjoy.

Considering and coming to terms with death, to the degree that anyone can, is an important—I say essential—part of life. It is only via this process that we can move forward. Without an awareness of your own demise it's easy to waste your time. And that's what most people in the Western world do with their lives: fill in the time between birth and death with distractions.

18

Walking home after dropping my son at school this morning, I realised that my safety issue is 'me feeling safe to be me'. This is the name I've given to a group of feelings that have been around for a long time but until now were unrecognised and unnamed. There's the slight panic at the thought of meeting a group of people I don't know. This manifests itself as an uneasiness in the area between my belly button and my chest (in my solar plexus) and I feel slightly sick. There's the fear of telling my parents bad news about myself, e.g. a relationship break-up. Here there is a tightening of my chest and a sensitisation of my throat so that it's almost sore and there's almost a lump in it. And then there's the fear of standing in the school playground waiting to pick my son up from school. I don't know what this feels like because, believing I cannot escape the task, I've resigned myself to it and have over-ridden my body's messages.

Because most of you will not share my fears, focusing on their specific nature will only separate you from me and create distance between us. Instead, focus on what underlies these fears, i.e. having an environment where it is safe for me to be me or, in your case, safe for you to be you. For me this book is the ultimate place of safety. It gives me the opportunity to say what I believe, in the manner I choose, without fear of interruption or contradiction. And this is important—indeed essential—for me because I can be unduly influenced by others, speaking not from my truth but to what the other person wants to hear. And when it comes to cancer, most people don't want to hear what I've got to say.

Do you want to hear: "You should have seen it coming. Or at least have been aware it was a real possibility"? Do you want to hear: "Your way of life is unsustainable and you have to change"? Do you want to hear: "You might die"? I doubt it. It's more likely that you want your view of life confirmed. To hear that everything will be OK, you'll live happily ever after and you won't have to change a thing... and that you'll win the lottery so you'll never have to work again!

Yes, what we want certainly *does* get in the way of the truth. And that is no less true for me than it is for you. Just under the surface, hidden until revealed by that last sentence, is a desire to get to the end of this book without doing the things I must do if I am to get to the end of it. But that's part of this book's magic. It's not only a set of thoughts on a page. It's not only a story waiting to be told. It is, for the duration of its writing, both my path and the light that illuminates it. And, as I said before, it's the thing that keeps me safe.

Thus it's like the rope in Nightline, a game I played on an adventure holiday in the Shropshire countryside. It involved walking blindfold through a wood, guided only by a rope and instructions from the person ahead. As the head of my group I led the rest of the party, feeling my way along the path and describing it to the person behind, with them in turn giving a description to the next in line.

Of all the activities it was Nightline and the trapeze I enjoyed most and, ironically, it was these I feared most before starting. What changed my mind about—or rather my bodily response to—both activities was the fact they were safe. For the trapeze I was supported on a safety wire with a breaking strain of eight tonnes and with Nightline, I knew the instructors would not lead us (via the rope) down a sheer ten-foot drop or through brambles. And should anything untoward happen—they did mention carnivorous squirrels (which was a joke on their part, in case any of you unfamiliar with the Shropshire countryside are in any doubt!)—the instructors were on hand and watched our progress every step of the way.

So, when half way up the telegraph pole on route to the trapeze, I was overcome not by fear, but by a fit of the giggles. It was such a ridiculous thing to do! Climb up a pole in the middle of the woods, only to jump from the top and hang swinging from a bar for a while. And with Nightline, once I had my hand on the rope, it was both easy going and enjoyable. The key was to be careful: to take small exploratory steps, test the ground for low obstacles and inclines, and move my free hand around my head and in front of my face to check for low branches and other dangers. As a result I got through Nightline completely unscathed and it was only when the activity ended and I took my blindfold off that I hit my head on a tree!

What does that say? Maybe that I—indeed we—rely too much on our sight, and that it is fallible. Or to put it another way, we believe what we see, but do not see everything. And the magic of this book is that it reveals to me—and to you—that which was previously hidden.

19

I wrote something yesterday and put it on my pin-board: "Without an acknowledgement and acceptance of all that we are, how can we be fully ourselves?" The answer is: We can't. Yet isn't this what we try to do? When there are bits of ourselves we don't like, we hide them and pretend they're not there. When there are elements of our past we'd rather forget, we bury them deep within ourselves hoping they'll disappear. And when there are parts of life we'd rather not face up to, we pretend that life is other than it is. This is our way. And it is the way of our bodies to counter this process using whatever means available: cancer included. Why do our bodies 'go wrong?' Because we have 'gone wrong', i.e. moved away from our true path. And the further we are from our path and the more we resist moving back to it, the bigger are the steps our bodies take away from health.

Only yesterday did I begin to see myself as I truly am. I thought I'd seen this person as a result of experiencing cancer, but I was wrong. Back then I saw only part of the picture—the best part. Before cancer the true me was completely hidden. I was out of touch with her and had forgotten she existed. Then along came something with such amazing strength and power that it pushed away the fears and insecurities that had come to define me, and let the true me emerge and breathe again. As cancer subsided my task became—it still is—to keep in touch with the true me, whilst allowing my fears and insecurities to reappear so that I can deal with them once and for all. Yesterday I saw that a number of these fears and insecurities still exist.

They are part of me and will continue to be so until I deal with them. To deny them or hope that they'll disappear is denying the truth and therefore denying who I am.

20

When I decided to write this book many people were horrified. It wasn't the writing that inspired this reaction but the giving up of my job and, in particular, the selling of my house:

"Surely there must be another way!?"

"Wait 'til you've paid off the mortgage!"

"You'll never get back on the housing ladder!"

"You've worked so hard to get where you are!"

"What happens when the money runs out?"

"What if the book doesn't get published?"

People couldn't get their heads round the fact that I was giving up my home to live in rented accommodation when conventional wisdom dictated that everybody should be aiming to own a house...and the bigger the house the better! I remember a conversation with a friend's husband that went something like this:

"But isn't the rent more than the mortgage?"

"Yes."

"So why are you selling your house?"

"Because it allows me to do what I want to do."

"But isn't the rent more than the mortgage?"

"Yes."

"So...so...why are you selling your house?"

"Because..."

And because we were talking after an all-day party and he'd had more than a few beers, the conversation went round like this not once or twice but at least six times until I could stand it no longer—my own laughter, that is! Even when stone-cold sober this guy couldn't get his head round the idea that anyone would move from their own home into rented accommodation and in the process double their housing costs.

To avoid such conversations now, I say, "I've bought my life back". This works in that people are more able to grasp and accept the motivation behind my decision. But to use the word "decision" is wrong. I didn't 'decide', i.e. 'make up my mind' to sell my house, instead I knew it was the right thing to do—knew in my body, not in my head. In my head of course this action didn't make sense—and it still doesn't, not that I'd thought about it until now. You see I stopped worrying whether my actions make sense a while ago. When I got cancer, to be exact.

Reacting to cancer as I did does not make sense from a conventional point of view—I admit it—but that doesn't make it wrong either. None of the things that take life out of the mundane and the ordinary make sense, do they? Think about it. Find the sense in the following: falling in love; the enjoyment in driving a fast car; the drive to create; having children; what makes you laugh.

Let's start with children. They don't make sense from a financial perspective as until they're 18 (and the rest!) all you do is pay out. Emotionally you give out too. You may be lucky enough to get something back but there are no guarantees. Although you share some of the same genes, you and your child may be completely different, indeed incompatible, and maybe you'll never understand him or her and vice versa. Having children has nothing to do with good sense and everything to do with the body. Either your body gets itself (or your girlfriend's self) pregnant without a thought from you (and I'm not talking forgetting to use contraception), or you decide to get pregnant out of some biological need. The desire to have children is not an intellectual thing. It exists in your body, not in your brain.

It's the same with falling in love. You can fall in love with someone's mind, but falling in love has nothing to do with the mind itself and everything to do with the body. If you're lucky enough to have experienced love, tap into that love now. What you get is a feeling in your body, probably in your heart chakra, perhaps in your tummy, perhaps somewhere else, but it's a feeling you get not a thought in your head. Any thoughts are something else. They are not the experience of love. You have no control over love. You can choose not to let it control you, but you can't stop loving just because you want to. Love has nothing to do with the mind and everything to do with the body.

And it's the same with the other things too. While intellect plays a part in driving, the enjoyment of a fast car comes from how it makes you feel. If you asked one hundred fast-car owners why they chose their vehicle, I don't think many would say, "because it was the sensible thing to do". Neither does what each of us finds funny make sense. Some of us may prefer intellectual jokes, while others prefer toilet humour, but laughter is a bodily not an intellectual response. It's hard to make yourself laugh and you certainly can't stop laughing just because you want to. Have you laughed at an inappropriate time? Or cried with laughter? Nothing can stop that save for your body and it only does so when it's ready to.

And finally the desire to create. I've left this 'til last because it's more complex. The need to create is biological, akin to the desire to have children. It comes out of the body, but with creativity it may not appear to be that way. Have you had a thought that seems to come out of nowhere such as, "I'll bake some cakes"? When such a thought does not follow a cookery programme on TV, or precede a visit from the grandchildren, or another trigger, it's created in response to an undetected signal from the body and is, therefore, your body leading the way. And in that way it's like cancer. Although what we have in these two cases are communications at either end of the body's range.

21

By now you should have an insight into the role of your body and awareness that, in some areas, your body is already in charge. It's getting you to take the next step that's difficult, i.e. giving yourself over to your body in all areas, including what you stand for, where you put your energies and the direction you take in life. But then again, you don't have a choice in the matter. If you don't do it voluntarily by listening to your body's subtle forms of guidance, before you know it your body takes charge in other ways—ways that include cancer.

To help with this I'll talk about what motivates the body to communicate and what it's trying to achieve, but before that I need to talk about what the body is. Your body is a compass. You can use it to find your way in the world. It can tell you which is the right way and which is the wrong way. And it can help you find your way back to your path when you are lost.

The difficulty in letting your body guide is in trusting that it's right when often it points you in a direction you are reluctant—if not unwilling—to go. I still struggle with this, even with everything I've experienced and everything I know. But this will always be the case because our bodies demand that we push at the interface between reality and delusion. And however much we know and however far we have come, that barrier will always exist because it moves with us.

But however true that is, you probably need more—something you can relate to and that will inspire you to let your body lead. The event that springs to mind took place last summer, about nine months ago, and is significant because it marks the first time I consciously acted on my body's more subtle communications concerning the right and the wrong way, and what it means to do so.

I was dating a man at the time, my last boyfriend. The relationship lasted six months and this event occurred around two months in. My boyfriend was planning a trip to the Isle of Man Grand Prix to see a friend race for the first time. He asked if I wanted to go with him. In the past I wouldn't have hesitated in saying yes. I'd not been to the Isle of Man and wanted to visit the island. I also wanted to spend time with my boyfriend. Plus, I had the weekend free and was pretty sure my parents would look after my son. Everything pointed to me going apart from one thing—it didn't feel right to do so.

When I asked myself if I should go the answer my body gave was no. It wasn't a strong no, it was subtle, but it was definitely no: a no in the area between my belly button and my heart in the form of a darkening and heaviness; a yes being the opposite of this, a lightness. What was significant about this 'no' was a) that I recognised it clearly and b) the contrast between it and my other thoughts and feelings. Whichever way I looked at it the signs pointed to me going and yet my body was telling me this was not the right thing to do. Maybe because of this very contrast, and certainly because the no feeling was clear, I told my boyfriend I wasn't going with him with no justification other than "it didn't feel right". He was OK about it, although he didn't understand, but it's not the impact of my decision on him that is important but how it affected me.

I didn't know what to expect when I said no. I knew only that this was what my body wanted me to do and that as I'd invested so much in this path, e.g. selling my house, I had to follow. If I didn't, everything would have been in vain. And that's the benefit of taking big steps, or big risks if that's how you'd prefer to describe them, for the bigger the step the easier it is to take all the little steps that follow and that are, in reality, much harder to take.

After the no came awareness—an awareness of what it meant to be on my path—and accompanying this was emotion, both panic and sorrow. I could see that in choosing to follow the no from my body I was choosing a path that may take me away from the man I was seeing; that if push came to shove, I'd choose my path over him. It was scary to be in that position—I liked my boyfriend and didn't want the relationship to end—but it was more than that too. Before that time I'd seen my path only in terms of success (e.g. publication of the book) or failure. But this was different. This was a marking out of the way.

And what a way! (I've resisted that link for a long time but really can't think of another way to get to this next bit, so sorry.) Because, as the panic and the sorrow subsided, I was left with a feeling of security I'd not felt before. Not the artificial security that comes from having a job, owning your own home or being in a relationship—because however much you *don't* want to face up to it, all these things could be taken from you—but the real security that comes from being true to yourself. And while you can give that away for sure, ain't no-one gonna take it from ya.

How this security manifested itself for me was in the context of relationships. In being prepared to choose my path over a relationship, I took away the ability of someone to hurt me to any large extent. Before I made that choice it was as if I was, figuratively speaking, floating around from place to place with no home other than when I was in a relationship when my home became his. This made me vulnerable to the whims of my partner and devastated when the relationship finished.

By choosing my path above and beyond all other things I grounded myself, giving myself a home and somewhere to come back to in those times outside of relationships. Thus, while the ending of a relationship can upset me to some extent (assuming I am emotionally engaged with it), I can never be hurt as deeply as I have been in the past.

22

It is fundamental to your mental, physical, emotional and spiritual health that you feel safe to be you. Sadly, this feeling eludes most of us for most of our lives. Not knowing how to spell "eludes" I looked it up in the dictionary and came across "illude" which means to trick. And that's what we do, illude—or indeed delude—ourselves that we're safe when in reality we're covering up the fact that we're not.

This goes back to the issue I touched on in the last chapter: the artificial security that comes from having a job, owning your own home or being in a relationship. While these are good and worthy goals, they're no replacement for the security that comes from being your own person, i.e. being true to yourself. We just kid ourselves they are. And my current task is to reveal that to you. Not to tell you—I've done that—but reveal it to you so that you *know*—with your body not with your head.

A good place to begin is with one of the central themes of this book: cancer. And how I've been taken back to this place by one of life's gifts. On the way to school this morning one of the dads gave me a book. In our occasional strolls between the school gate and pedestrian crossing (about a five-minute walk) I've been talking to him about my book. The book he gave me was another woman's breast cancer story: *Journeys (with a Cancer)* by Jenny Cole. He'd seen it on a second-hand bookstall and thought of me—which was sweet, wasn't it?

I looked at the book on my walk home then put it on a shelf in my office not knowing what it was for. When I reached the end of the last section I didn't know how to reveal to you the truth of the security myth, then I saw this book. Being me I thought, "maybe the next part of the puzzle will be revealed by that book", and took it off the shelf and opened it at random. The page on the left revealed nothing but the page on the right revealed two sentences: "We talked of security, and how I didn't have any", and further down the page, "I felt so safe with him".

I read through the first sentence without consciously registering it and needed to be alerted to it by a wobbly feeling in my body. Imagine a wave starting at the base of your torso and moving up to your head causing you to move backwards then forwards as it goes—it was that kind of wobbly feeling. As the wave got to neck height my brain finally registered what my body had seen and said, "wait a minute, what was that?!" or something similar, and it was then that I looked back at the sentence.

I could scour the entire book looking for other places where the words safety and security appear on the same page but I can't be bothered (no offence Jenny), and a statistical analysis to determine the likelihood of finding those two words on a page is not what's needed here. But for those of you who do need something along these lines, I worked back through the book, opening it about ten times, every ten to twenty pages or so, and skim read it for those two words. I found neither. These issues do not appear to be key words in the book. And even if those words did appear often in the book, so what? It's not only that I found those two words on the same page at a random opening of the book that's amazing, but that I had the book to open in the first place and that it had been given to me only this morning.

I say 'amazing', but it's not—this kind of thing happens to me all the time. It must do or why would I think, "maybe the next part of the puzzle will be revealed to me by that book?" Any person basing their lives on sense or logic—perish the thought!—wouldn't think this way, would they? But I *do* think this way. Why? Because I know from experience that life works this way if you allow it to. If you're in touch with the true you and come from that place, not only do you have at your disposal the wisdom of your body but you tap into the very essence of life itself. And when you do that truly amazing things do happen, things that put my experience with the cancer book into the shade.

I'm drawn to tell you of the day before my mastectomy. I need to tell this story now because that day was one of the most amazing days of my life so far. It's one of only two days when my body has spoken to me in words—yes, words from my body and not from my head—and it's also the day when life gave me the clearest possible messages as to which way I should go.

I had an appointment with my surgeon that morning. It was the first time I'd seen him since cancelling my planned mastectomy on the day it should have taken place the month before. (I'll tell you more about the decision to cancel later in the book.) Owing to holiday commitments, the surgeon could operate only the next morning or in two weeks time. As eleven weeks had passed since the initial diagnosis and the cancer was growing rapidly—from a pea to a plum to a tangerine in just under three months—both the surgeon and the breast-care nurse advised me to have the operation as soon as possible.

Sharing their concerns I booked the operation for the next day but still had doubts that this was the right thing to do, arising out of the few bits of me that had not accepted a mastectomy as the only way forward. I left the hospital asking for a sign that I'd be right to have the operation sooner rather than later. I had a car that day and drove from the hospital to my son's nursery. Leaving the city on the ring-road I heard a song on the radio that hinted at the next day being right for the operation, but the lyrics were ambiguous and the doubts in my mind were stronger and overrode them.

Realising this was not good enough I asked for another sign—or rather, I pleaded. Had my hands not been on the steering wheel and my eyes upon the road, both would have been raised to the heavens as indications of the strength of my call. Pulling up outside the nursery I saw one next-day delivery van parked on the verge and as I got out of the car another passed by. While for some of you these may have been sufficient to say, "Yes! I'm right to have the operation tomorrow", for me they began only to dissipate my doubts. It was as if they drew my attention to the possibility of clear signs without me registering them as such. They were enough to raise my awareness slightly, so opening my eyes and ears for what was to follow.

I had to go into the nursery to pick up my son. As it was open from 8 a.m. 'til 6 p.m. parents could collect their children at any time and I had to wait for him to stop what he was doing and get ready for home. The children were painting that day and easels stood to my right displaying the morning's work. To protect the easels from the worst of the paint and to provide a dry base for the paper they had first been covered with newspaper some of which was visible around the edges of the pictures.

Two headlines on the easel closest to me caught my eye. I'd be lying if I said I can remember exactly what the headlines said, I can't. But I can remember their tone and the fact that unlike the lyrics of the song they were not open to interpretation. They leapt up at me from the newsprint demanding my attention. "URGENT ACTION REQUIRED!" and "THE TIME IS RIGHT!" or, as I've explained, something very similar. Although I don't think I took a step back on reading those headlines I could well have done, and even if I didn't respond outwardly something changed in me on reading them. Before registering their words I desperately wanted a sign and was searching for one. As I read them I opened up to the possibility that the signs were there. Life was speaking to me. Life was showing me the way.

The experience left me slightly dazed, as you'd expect from a shift in perception—think drugs without the drugs—and I left the nursery, son in hand, not quite of this world. Getting into the car to set off for home my fate was sealed. Another two next-day delivery vans passed by, four in the space of five or so minutes. Too many, too close together, to be ignored. Driving home I already knew, at a bodily level, that the operation had to be the next day, but my thinking took longer to catch up. Even though the doubts had been pushed aside by the clear signs I'd been given, I wasn't at the point where I wanted to have the operation. It's not that I didn't want it—that feeling had passed—but having spent so long not wanting it, I was still influenced by that feeling.

When I got home I sat on the sofa; I believe I still had my jacket on and my car keys in my hand. Nothing in particular was going through my mind, and I certainly wasn't running through my experiences in my head. Instead, I was being with the things I'd seen and allowing myself to absorb them. After I'd sat for ten or twenty seconds, a minute at the very most, I heard and felt the following words: "We can't hold this off much longer." And this time that is *exactly* what was said.

You know that place I refer to? The one between the belly button and the heart? That's where the words came from. They rose from there to meet my consciousness and were, therefore, words of the body. They were not—I am absolutely positive—thoughts in my head. How do I know this? Believe me, I *know* what the voice in my head sounds like. As I said way back in Chapter 1, it used to be that the constant hum of my thoughts was the background noise to my life. And even though I don't think half as much as I used to I still think a lot, especially when I'm a little lost.

How many thoughts does a person have in a day? 10? 50? 100? 250? I don't know, but it's a lot. For the purpose of this story let's be conservative and say 100. I'm sure it's more than this but I want to choose a number on the low side so you don't think I'm overestimating and get caught up in that. If you think 100 is an overestimate, consider this. With sixteen waking hours a day, that's eight hours sleep a night, you need only three thoughts an hour to generate 48 thoughts a day; just six thoughts an hour and you have 96. So 100 thoughts a day is about one thought every ten minutes. That's nothing, is it? Thus, as a thirty-nine year old, I've easily had one million thoughts in my head. (That's less than 28 years worth[13]).

So when I heard the words, "we can't hold this off much longer", I had the sound of at least one million thoughts to compare it with. Plenty enough to build up a wealth of experience, wouldn't you say? And trust me, it was *not* the same. For a start it sounded different. Say something in your head then say it again out loud; then get someone else to say the same thing. Although the same words are being said each time, the experience of hearing these words isn't the same, is it? It's easy to distinguish between them, isn't it? When the words rose up from that place between my belly button and my heart, it was obvious they were coming from my body and not from my head. I could hear it and I could feel it too.

You know what happens when you hit a drum? The skin vibrates, the air around it vibrates and the air carries the sound to your eardrum, which then vibrates so you can hear the sound? When my body spoke the words, "we can't hold this off much longer", I could also feel a vibration. It started in the centre of me and moved out through my body in all directions. But although the words were spoken what I felt wasn't a sound vibration, it was energy—which, when it comes down to it, is all vibration is.

23

That's the story of my body (and life) speaking to me in words. The words from my body were real—I'm not making it up!—and I've done my best to demonstrate that I can tell the difference between these and my thoughts given that I've spent a lifetime listening to myself chattering in my head; so whether or not you believe my story is up to you.

I'm saying this because I'm pretty sure some of you won't believe it. Either you won't believe it's possible for my body to speak or you'll think that, despite my protestations, I'm making it up. To those who fit that description I'll say this: "I'm sorry. There's nothing I can do about it. I'm going to move on." Something I realised only recently and that was brought home to me clearly yesterday is that I can only speak my truth. What you do with it is up to you.

Where I've been wrong in the past is in thinking that if someone doesn't get 'it', it's something to do with me and how I've put it across. In reality it's more likely something in the other person that stops them seeing it, maybe that they don't want to. To help explain this I'll tell you what happened yesterday. Yet another example of life giving me what I need, when I need it.

I was in the park with my son. It was after school and late, in what had been an enjoyably warm afternoon. A woman came into the children's play area with her toddler son and a black Labrador dog...It's the next bit I'm struggling with. I know—in my body, not in my head—that it's important for me to try—although I'm not sure why—to communicate the subtle changes that occurred in me and that resulted in me talking to the woman about her dog. A key point is that the changes happened gradually over the preceding month, thus what happened in the park was the culmination of something.

It's also important that you understand my motivation and emotional state, because the changes relate to what I was trying to achieve when I spoke to the woman and how I felt about it. Dogs are not allowed in the park and I talked to the woman about this. As I wasn't sure whether the rule applied to the whole park or only to the kiddies play area, I checked on a sign at the entrance to the park before speaking to her. Looking back I can see that the conversation with the woman was different because a) I had it whereas in the past I would have been too fearful to do so, and b) despite having been so afraid for so long, I was not afraid to speak to her. Although I was careful in approaching her, e.g. checking my facts and speaking in a calm voice (at least initially), I wasn't 'afraid' of what she might say or 'afraid' of what she might do. And I certainly wasn't afraid of what she might think, which is something that has held me back for years.

The other difference was my motivation. If you'd asked, as I approached the woman, why I wanted to speak to her, I would have said: "Because dogs are not allowed in the park."

"We know that!" I hear you cry. "You've told us!"

Yes, but the important thing here is that I wanted to talk to her *only* because dogs are not allowed and she had her dog with her, and not for any other purpose, e.g. I didn't want her to remove the dog. It's important that you see and understand this difference because it's easy to mistake speaking your truth with getting what you want and these things are *not* the same at all—and more about this later in the book, I'm sure! The conversation went something like this:

"Did you know dogs aren't allowed in the park?"

"Isn't it just the play area?"

"No, it's the whole park and anyhow your dog *is* in the play area."

"I'll just be a few minutes and then I'll go."

"OK," I said and walked away. When the woman was still in the park five minutes later, I spoke to her again. (This is the gist of the conversation. More was said but these are the key points.)

"You're still here with your dog and you said you'd leave."

"I've made the effort to come out. I'm here with my son. I'll go soon."

"Dogs are not allowed in the park."

"What business is it of yours what I do!?"

"You've brought your dog into this public space where dogs are not allowed and I'm here with my son, so it *is* my business. Now it looks as if your dog is going to be sick and that's disgusting! He could have weed or pooed anywhere and kids play here."

"I know he hasn't done anything."

"No you don't! You've not been watching him all the time. How do you know?"

"Look! What's it got to do with you? I've made the effort to come out. I'm here with my son. I'll go in a few minutes. I won't bring the dog back. What more do you want?"

At that point I collected my son and walked home. I don't know when the woman left. And the point of the story? I'm not sure! No, that's not right. I am sure but I can't see why it fits in now. But as it feels right it must be right.

By not having an agenda when I spoke to the woman, i.e. not wanting anything from the conversation, what I got from the conversation—ha!—was to see the woman as she truly was, in that situation and at that time: someone who was prepared to break the rules, albeit just for a little while, to get what she wanted. Or to put it another way, she wasn't prepared to see 'it'—it being the absolute that dogs are not allowed in the park—because she had something to lose by doing so. Ah! *That's* where it fits in. And so the question becomes:

What do you have to lose by not seeing things my way? (Not that I want you to, of course!)

24

Let's turn our attention back to cancer and focus on why your body gave it to you. If I've communicated effectively and you've been paying attention, this is what you'll have picked up so far: your body gave you cancer to communicate something; part of the message is you've forgotten who you are; and don't get hung up on death because it's a side issue. It's this last point I need to talk about now because unless you see cancer for what it isn't, you'll never be able to see it for what it is.

A few days ago I realised I'm no longer afraid to talk about death. I didn't have a breakthrough in thinking, instead something shifted inside me taking the fear with it. After the story of the woman and her dog I can see what's happened. I've let go of wanting to achieve a specific outcome—or rather wanting to avoid one, i.e. upsetting you—and in so doing have let go of the fear of speaking my truth about death. Now I can see that—just like the woman and her dog—any problems you have with death come from you and not from me. If you don't want to face up to death that's your problem and not mine—because die you will at some point.

Like many people, I'd taken on board the taboo that society has around death and made it my own. People are afraid to talk about death because they're afraid to die, and not talking about it means they can forget about it for a while. The problem with this strategy is that when the time comes and you *have* to face up to death, you're not ready—hence much upset and hand-wringing. And it's this I need to talk about now. You may think "upset and hand-wringing" is rather a dismissive phrase to describe the feelings that accompany coming to terms with death. I don't. I feel this way because, while some feelings that accompany a possible or probable death are genuine, most are a way of avoiding facing up to it. There, I've said it. This is my opening line and you're the woman in the park. How will you react? The woman in the park was aggressive. Is that how you're going to be?

This is an issue of responsibility. The woman owned the dog: she was responsible for it being in the park. This is your life: you are responsible for it both now and at the end, i.e. in death. Being a human being *does* bring with it responsibilities that are there whether you want to face up to them or not.

The woman chose to ignore the no-dogs rule because she didn't want to obey it; she thought she'd lose something by doing so. And in the way we live our lives in the West, we too are choosing to ignore the rules by which we should live. So much so, and so widely, we no longer know what they are. We too believe that we'll lose something if we follow them. In fact we, like the woman, have nothing to lose and everything to gain.

The rules that govern us are not written on signs or tablets of stone. They are part of us. We cannot read these rules and follow them through our intellect, instead we are made aware of them by our bodies. Using sensation and emotion our bodies tell us when we are aligned with our rules—our truth—and when our behaviour is out of line. But because it is with emotion and sensation that our bodies communicate with us, we have taken to using these against the body when it says something we don't want to hear. We do this with people too.

The woman in the park didn't want to hear: "Dogs are not allowed in the park". To stop hearing this, i.e. to stop me saying it, she tried using emotion, i.e. she got angry and aggressive. She tried to make it my problem and not hers: "what's it got to do with you?" And she tried to justify what she was doing: "I've made the effort to come out. I'm here with my son. I'll go in a few minutes."

What did you do in response to the following? "While some feelings that accompany a possible or probable death are genuine, most are a way of avoiding facing up to it." Did you use emotion, e.g. get angry and aggressive? Did you try to make it my problem? "She's got a cheek! What does she know about it? Who is she to tell me what to think?" Or did you try to justify what you do when you get upset about death? "I've only just heard I have cancer! I might die! I'm going to die!"

To help with this—it *is* a difficult thing to come to terms with and sometimes even to grasp—I'm going to share with you my breakthrough moment about death. It happened one evening in the weeks following diagnosis when I was lying in bed thinking about, or rather fearing, death. Yes, I did do this. And not only does it fit with the text for me to share this with you now, it's important that I do so in order that your picture of me continues to become more rounded.

Because my message is so different from the conventional view of cancer and death—"What a terrible thing! How sad! How young they are! Life is so unfair! Why me?/Why you?/Why them?/Why us?/Why now?"—I run the risk of creating a divide between us; of you seeing me as different from you: stronger than you, braver than you, madder than you, or however it is that you define and measure the perceived differences between us. I know this is a real possibility—in my body *and* in my head—and that's why I've written this book in the way that I have. What I have to say cannot be said quickly or with only a few words.

But sometimes, because of the very nature of the path, I need to be more forceful with you. Some of what you see and hear will be (has been) shocking. It will scare you and you will be afraid. And because of this you'll not want to carry on with me. You'll want to turn back and return to the comfort of the place you came from. The place you believe to be safe. But—and it's important that you hear this—that place is not safe. Whatever its outside appearance, however much you believe it to be safe, it is not. It cannot be safe because that place gave you cancer.

25

My head, my hands, my legs, my feet are still
Laid out by fear
My mind is channel-hopping
One image follows the next
The cancer is spreading
From breast to lymph
From lymph to liver
From liver to lung
My body is eating itself from the inside
An exponential decay

Each heartbeat drums out the march of death
But still it arrives suddenly
Dark and suffocating
A motherless child stands alone beside an empty bed
A funeral gathers, weeps and dissipates

But then change
Suddenly only my torso seems to exist
I have no limbs, no head or neck
All of my weight and all of my consciousness
Inhabit the trunk of my body
The weight of my existence focuses itself
In one place
In one moment of time
And I can see

Even if I live until I'm seventy
I'll still not be ready to die
I'm living a life that has little to do with the true me
To all intents and purposes
I am dead
Already

This is what we avoid seeing when we avoid facing up to death. It's not death we are afraid of but seeing our lives in the *context* of death. Death is a huge light that shines down on us revealing the full landscape of our lives, opening up the dark corners and hidden crevices to full view. In the face of death—faced with the truth of our lives—we can no longer hide from who we are and what we have done. Unless, of course, this is the path we choose.

To help with this let's go back to the woman in the park. Think of death as the park warden who finds the woman with her dog. There's no point getting angry and aggressive with him because that's not going to get you off, is it? There's no point proclaiming: "What business is it of yours?" For it is the job of the park warden, just as it is death's job, to call us to account. And there's no point trying to justify why you broke the rules or argue that you didn't know about them, because if you take the trouble to look, the rules are clearly laid out for you to follow.

So, faced with the park warden what does the woman do? My guess is she'll be sorry and, if it is her way, she'll shed some tears. She'll apologise to the park warden for breaking the rules and, if it is her way, she'll tell him she didn't know of the no-dog rule. If she's lucky, the park warden will let her off with a warning and obediently the woman will leave the park, grateful to the warden for letting her off this time.

It's what she does on the way home, after the crisis is over, that determines the impact of this event on her life. If it is her way, she'll start to feel pleased with herself and how she 'got away with it'. She'll smile at how she lied so convincingly to the park warden and boast about it to her husband and friends later in the day. She'll be slightly surprised that she cried when first confronted by the warden, but will dismiss this as hormonal, or stress, or tiredness. And, if it is her way, she'll think about the other woman in the park—that busy body!—and assume that she called the warden. The incident will become the other woman's fault and she will be the victim.

If this is how the woman deals with the event it will have little impact on her life, other than to dig her deeper into it. It will not change what she thinks. It will not change how she reacts in the future. It will not make her question who she is and who she's being. It will be simply something that happened to her, an example of life getting in the way and something to be forgotten.

And isn't this how we'd all like it to be—cancer, that is? We want to 'get away with it', having gone through only a little pain and having shed only a few tears. We want to move away from it as quickly as possible and consign it to the past. We want to forget about it and get on with our lives. Yes, what we want is 'business as usual'. We may take a few obvious lessons away with us—for the woman in the park, don't bring your dog with you; for the cancer patient, eat a better diet, give up smoking and reduce stress levels—but we don't really want to look at what's underneath it all. What got us here in the first place and where we should go next.

I say "we" because that's how I was when I found out I had cancer. Yes, there was the euphoria—knowing that this was the thing that would sort my life out—but underneath that I was the same as you. There was a huge resistance to change and to seeing things as they truly are. How that manifested in me is different to the way it manifests in you because we are different. We are different people with different life experiences. But that doesn't mean you can't learn from me and it doesn't mean I can't learn from you: look at what the woman in the park has shown me. And what you need to do now is to believe that I have something to teach you and that you are able to learn. Put aside your doubts and trust in me; look past the fear of death to what is on the other side; for it is there that the path begins.

PART FOUR

26

I sometimes say 13 is my lucky number. I'm not sure that it is but I'm certainly not afraid of it, living at a number 13 as I do. I think I claim 13 as my lucky number because of the impact it has on people. It says, "there's something different about this woman"—to some people, something not normal! I've realised in the past few weeks that I do this a lot, the 'not normal' thing. There's selling my house to write a book, giving up alcohol, the 'can't eat anything that normal people eat' diet and, of course, the way I reacted to cancer. All these actions signal that there's something different about me.

I'm not sure whether I do these things because I'm different, or because it's only by doing these things that I can be different—if there is a difference between those two things—and it doesn't matter which it is. What's important is the freedom I get from being this way. It's so incredibly difficult to be different in this world; the pressure to conform is enormous. But in this way it's like atmospheric pressure: we've grown up with it, we live with it and we get on with our lives in the presence of it. Quite simply, we're used to it. However, whereas we need atmospheric pressure to survive because our bodies have evolved under its influence, this is not the case with other pressures upon us. However, these pressures have made us who we are.

We are two people, you and I. By that, I don't mean that you are separate from me—although you are while we are both of this earth—but that each of our personalities, as expressed though our actions, has one of two sources. There is the 'true you' and there is the 'other you'. The true you is your unique spiritual identity expressed in human form. The true you is eternal. It is your soul. It is the little bit of you that is God. The other you is the 'stuff' that covers up the true you. The other you does not exist when you are born but is created via your experiences and the influence of others, including your family, society and culture.

The person writing this book is the true me. Sometimes the other me creeps in, mainly via my fears and insecurities, but mostly I keep this person at bay. And it is because I can do this more easily in this forum than in any other area, that this book is so important to me.

With practice, and knowing what to look for, you can learn to distinguish the true from the other you. But to do this you need to know what it feels like to be each person—and that's where the problem is. Many of us are cut off from our true selves to such a large extent we've forgotten this person exists—it was certainly that way for me before I had cancer—and because of this we spend most of our lives living as the other person. Or, to put it another way, we spend most of our lives living *someone else's* life.

27

If I'd talked about my childhood before now, I'd have given you the wrong information. You'd have become caught up in my version of my life story, just as I've been caught up in it most of my life. What I'd have told you wouldn't have been true. Ironically, the fairy tale in Chapter 3 is the true version of my life and what I've believed until now is fiction, i.e. made-up.

Before we move onto my early life — the days long before divorce and cancer—I want to acknowledge how magical it is that I could put my hands on the truth, via the fairy tale, six months before it was known to my conscious self. And how, in so doing, I kept back this part of the book until I was ready to write it. How was that possible? I wrote the fairy tale because my body told me the book needed to go in that direction, and I ignored the parts of me that disagreed with this as the way forward. And when I wrote the fairy tale, I did so bypassing my head. I didn't think what to type but allowed the words to grow out of my body and through my fingertips, born of my true (or as Clarissa Pinkola Estés would put it, my wild) self.

The body is truly amazing, but for it to work as intended we need to believe in it and give it the space and freedom it needs.

When looking back at my childhood for clues as to why I was miserable for a long time, I thought my mum and dad were at fault. Now I can see that nobody is to blame.

They cared for me in the way they believed to be right but I, being me, needed something more. I was the little girl in the fairy tale, born into a family of giants but not being one at all. My parents were brought up in rural England, during the Second World War. Times were hard for everyone then but especially for my mum's family, being as large as it was. She was the second youngest of seven children—five boys above her and a sister below—and both food and clothes were hard to come by. She had to make do with hand-me-downs from other families in the village and having big feet (something I've inherited), the shoes did not fit well. The shape her toes make is a triangle rather than the quarter circle.

Why am I telling you this? Because I need to show her suffering and how this affected her relationship with her parents, or rather how it didn't. My mum was in no doubt that they loved her, despite her ill-fitting shoes. Everybody made sacrifices in those days and the sacrifices you made for your family were made out of love. But for me, born in 1965 and growing up in the 1960s and 1970s, I didn't see the sacrifices my mum and dad made in that way, indeed I didn't see them at all. I saw only that we didn't have a car, that we never went abroad and that, unlike the little girl over the road, my sister and I didn't have sweets every day.

But this isn't about the material things that were not there, but the emotional and spiritual vacuum in which we grew up. Mum and Dad were there for us in the way they thought they should be—putting food on the table, making sure we had a good education, keeping us on the straight and narrow, i.e. in the ways that were important to them and in their families when they were growing up—but I am not like them and I needed other things. And—this is what is so important—I didn't know it. Just like the little girl in the fairy tale, by the time I learnt to communicate with my parents I didn't know I wasn't the same as them. And because of that I had no choice but to grow up as one of them and try to fit in.

Looking at it now I can see there's something missing from the fairy tale: a middle section. Something after me growing up into a "giant to be proud of" but before I meet the other little girl in the woods who was, of course, the true me. There's nothing in the tale about my internal world and in particular the impact of growing up as someone else—someone other than the true me. From the point of view of this overall story—the story of how it is that cancer could transform my life and release the true me—this is probably the most important part. Perhaps its omission is symbolic of the fact that 'I', i.e. the true me, was missing during that time. As I'm not an expert on fairy tales I'm not going to dwell on this, but it's important that I tell you about my internal world for it is this, above and beyond anything else, that I needed saving from. But how do I do it so that it works for you?

The biggest problem I face, in writing this book, is getting you to the point where you can say, in all honesty: "Of course she reacted to cancer that way." Because if it becomes possible *in your eyes* for me to have had this experience, then such an experience also becomes possible for you. It's just a series of steps from where you are now to this other place.

Steps that you are capable of taking
Should the path be known.

28

To live life without the true you is to live an abiotic life, i.e. a life without life. I experienced this truth when I listened to my husband with my whole being, and again when I stepped out of the hospital into the sunshine the day the doctor told me I had cancer. And it is this that I saw and finally understood when I lay in bed thinking about death and realised that because I wasn't living a life based on the true me, I was dead already. In this last case it was through my own realisation that I stepped from one world into another, i.e. from that of the 'other' to the 'true' me. From this I can see that contrast is important, not just the darkness of one world and the light of another, but setting them beside each other so that each can be seen in the context of the other. It's also important that you understand cancer's role in this. How cancer was the wedge hammered between the two worlds and how I managed to keep it there for long enough to see them as separate, to firmly establish myself in the world of the true me and not slip back into the world of the other me as I'd done before.

I remember talking to a friend about an answer-phone message I left for her the day I was diagnosed. It included the phrase, "it's not a cyst, it's cancer". What surprised her was how I said this—as if what I had was less than, i.e. better than, the alternative; so much so that she thought she'd misheard me, "...it's not cancer, it's a cyst...". I remember leaving the message. It was the first call I made on my return from hospital. I'd spoken to my friend a few days before and was calling to get the number of her acupuncturist. Repeating the phrase, "it's not a cyst, it's cancer", I can see why my tone surprised her. It was the hint of relief in my voice. In hindsight, relief at having, at long last, something real to deal with.

My current counsellor was the first person to say, with complete understanding and conviction: "Of course you reacted that way to cancer." Her reasoning being that the cancer was real, whereas the things I'd struggled with prior to that were unreal. I'd spent all my life until I got cancer struggling with things that weren't real—and guess what happens when you do that? You can't win.

When something happens, you go one of three ways: you take it inside, i.e. you blame yourself; you project it outside, i.e. you blame someone else; or you see it for what it is and deal with it accordingly, laying blame where blame is due but learning from it and moving on. When I was growing up I took everything inside, and it is by this process that I started to create my imaginary world: the world of the other me.

It's going to be hard, this next bit, because part of you doesn't want to hear what I have to say. It's not like me 'enjoying cancer'—that behaviour is so unusual and so removed from your own that you can remain interested in it without being threatened by it. This is different. This is getting closer to the truth—for both me and for you—and that may be too close for comfort.

We all have an imaginary world: a way of being and of thinking that enables us to exist in this world without having to deal with the reality of it. We begin to create our imaginary world when we are children and, unless something comes along to get us out of it, it continues to grow to the point where it takes us over completely. The longer we inhabit our imaginary world and the deeper into it we fall, the harder it is to leave and the greater our resistance to doing so. There is, after all, much to be faced in stepping back into reality and there are also reasons why we left it in the first place. And, as all that is to be dealt with has to be dealt with if we are to leave the world of our imagination and make a full transition back to reality, it's not an easy thing to do.

The problem I have is getting you to accept that you are, in this respect, the same as everyone else. You have an imaginary world but you don't see it; you shy away from reality but don't believe it to be so. I've already touched on this though, with my discussion of cancer and how you reacted to it. Remember: you believed you might win the lottery jackpot—odds of 14 million-to-one—but you didn't think cancer—odds of three-to-one per lifetime—would happen to you. I'm not going to find a better example to highlight your two worlds and your preference as to which you inhabit—not without talking to you in person and that, given the medium of this story, is not a possibility. But this in itself is probably not enough. And although I can tell you things about yourself, this is not the same as discovering them on your own. So I need to turn my attention back to me and hope that in describing the two worlds I inhabit, you will see in them something of yourself.

29

In the imaginary world I created—the world of the other me—my mum and dad didn't love me. I knew this because they didn't kiss me, they didn't hug me and they didn't tell me of their love. And these were things that I, being me, needed to experience in order to feel—or to *be* in my other world—loved. This was my darkest secret; the keystone that held together my imaginary world. And this secret needed to leave the realm of the imaginary and be spoken in reality to make my transition to reality a permanent one.

I realise this may not make sense at the moment but by the end of the book it will. There are lots of threads to be pulled together and the best way for me to do this is to draw your attention to the knot, so to speak, before showing you how it was formed. Let's start with the window cleaner from Chapter 13. This story showed how to break free of the illusory world and step forward into reality simply by saying what's there.

I had little to lose by sharing my delusions with the window cleaner. Because he wanted to sell me his services he was duty bound to get on with me if he could, and if it did go horribly wrong I didn't have to see him again. But it's not always like that, is it? In most situations where we avoid speaking our truth—or what we believe to be our truth—we do so because we believe we've something to lose. While we're right to see that, we're wrong in what we think it is. All we have to lose are our delusions and our ability to stay in our illusory world. Believing we have anything else to lose is delusional.

I've said that, and I know it's right, but you may disagree. And that's what I'm up against. Or rather that's what *you're* up against, because it's not me who suffers from you living in your illusory world (not directly), it's you. This suffering holds the key to everything. Remember: I did all my suffering *before* I had cancer—and it's the contrast between the before and after that's so important here. I need to show you the extent of your suffering and reveal to you the cost of your delusory world. But you already know the cost of it: it's cancer. It's getting you to look back at your life to see it for what it really is, that's the challenge.

Before cancer I didn't know how important it was for me to speak to my mum and dad about feeling unloved. I say that, and it's true, but to say it in such a simple way belies the reality of living with this belief, day in and day out. Before I carry on with this however, I need to talk about the reality of living in an illusory world, which appears to be a contradiction but is not. What makes your world illusory are the thoughts in your head and the beliefs that you hold and the fact that these contradict reality. You still exist in the real world but you're not fully engaged with it because of the stuff in your head.

When living in an illusory world your body exists in reality but the world inside your body, as a result of the thoughts in your head, is unreal (illusory). Your body is the membrane between the two worlds and it is the energy flow between these worlds that engenders changes in your body. At first your body channels the energy flows and you experience these as sensation and emotion. If you don't change your internal world in response to these feelings you'll continue to experience them unless you suppress or repress them, but if you do this the energy acts on the body in a different way causing illness and disease.

Our bodies talk to us in the same way when we're living in reality: sensations and emotions are generated in response to energy flows between our internal and external worlds. In the crudest terms, therefore, living in an illusory world feels the same as living in reality because we experience it in the same way: through our bodies and via sensation and emotion. However, dig a little deeper and the two worlds and our experience of them could not be further apart.

Emotional pain and sorrow do not exist when living in reality. They are products of an illusory world. We feel these emotions only when we do not live in reality, accepting it for what it is. And it's the same with happiness and joy except the other way round. We cannot experience deep and lasting happiness and feel truly joyful when we're living in illusion. These emotions come from living in reality and it is through such emotions that our bodies show us we are there.

I know this is hard to understand but bear with me. My story of the time after diagnosis will help with this. Remember from the Preface: "Coming out of cancer, my goal has been to create a life where I can be as alive and as free as I was with cancer. I want to experience life as I did with cancer. I want to feel about life the way that I did with cancer". Cancer was the best time of my life because it was the most real. Cancer only looks bad from a place of illusion.

30

How was it living day in and day out with the belief that my mum and dad didn't love me? I don't know. Because I'd pushed that belief down inside me such a long time before, most of the time I wasn't aware it was there. And that's the hard part, isn't it? Getting you to see—as I had to see—things you don't want to see because they're too painful.

By taking a belief inside and hiding it, we seek to protect ourselves from the fallout from that belief—in my case the pain, and perhaps some shame, arising from the belief that my parents didn't love me. Because avoiding this pain and thus keeping the belief hidden becomes paramount, we do everything in our power to achieve this. We avoid all conversations and interactions that would give rise to the belief but in so doing stop the belief being tested. I didn't want to be reminded that my parents didn't love me so I avoided all situations that would show this to be the case. I withdrew from them so they could not withdraw from me. However, by adopting this approach I also avoided all situations that would reveal my belief to be untrue. I thus imprisoned myself within it.

I said before that when something happens, you go one of three ways: you take it inside (blame yourself); project it outside (blame someone else); or you see it for what it is and deal with it accordingly. With the first two you're creating an illusory world, with the last you're living in reality. The approach we choose in any given circumstance depends on that circumstance, the people involved and where we are emotionally and spiritually. It also depends on whether we're aware that we have a choice—most of us are not. We're all capable of taking any of the three paths but tend to prefer one path over the others: the one that works best for us. My childhood established my preferred path as taking it inside dealing with it there. This is why I retreated from my parents and didn't go at them all guns blazing—not until after cancer anyhow. Mum and Dad: sorry about that, I couldn't do anything else at the time.

By taking everything inside and dealing with it internally, the only way I could cope with the situations life threw at me was to adapt myself, or my view of the world, to fit what I saw. My (unconscious) reasoning was that the world was right and I was wrong and that I must change myself to fit. Thinking back to the fairy tale, I had forgotten I was not a giant and so had no choice but to become one—and a very good one I was too. I did well at school; I got a degree; I had a good job; I bought a house; I got married; I had a son. I did all the things that were expected of me; all the things that in the land of the giants were supposed to make me happy. But I wasn't happy—not truly happy, not deeply happy, not long time happy—happiness came in fits and starts but it was always fleeting and never satisfying to the soul.

Only when I listened to my husband with my whole being, and again when I recognised cancer as the thing that was going to save me, did I feel happiness that fills you from the inside out. Happiness that gives you that lightness of being, that buoyancy, that singing heart. Happiness that glows inside you like a fire and that brings tears of joy to your eyes. This happiness comes from embracing reality. This happiness comes from truth. This is happiness as it is *meant* to be experienced; as God intended it, if you like. And it is this happiness—and much, much more—that awaits you when you live life as the true you.

31

Now is a good time to talk about the other happiness: the happiness we use to escape from reality and to escape from truth. This covers you from the outside in but never quite gets to where it needs to be; it never quite hits the spot. And the reason it does this—or rather doesn't do this—is because it's there to silence the true you.

When living in an illusory world, i.e. when living as the other you, your body responds with negative sensations and emotions. These correspond to the energy differential between reality and your internal world. The bigger the difference, the bigger the negative emotions and the further you are from living life as the true you. Instead of dealing with the cause of these feelings, i.e. aligning ourselves with our truth, we mask the feelings with others. Why? Because it is easier. How? We do things to make ourselves feel better—we buy things; we go on holiday; we daydream; we get drunk—and while there is nothing inherently wrong with this behaviour, if you do it for the wrong reasons it *is* wrong for you.

This may be difficult to understand, as with other things in this book, so I'll help with a story. It's my friend's story though and I'm nervous about using it without her permission. In *Women Who Run with the Wolves*, Clarissa Pinkola Estés says that "gaining explicit permission to tell another's tale...is absolutely essential...It is a sign of respect...to ask and receive permission, [and] to not take work that has not been given freely...A story is not just a story. In its most innate and proper sense, it is someone's life." I need to go with the flow though so I'll tell the story and get permission later. (I did.)

My friend is an artist; she works mainly in clay. At Christmas she bought a mug from an art gallery. It was hand-made by another artist and cost £28. This, it must be said, is a lot for a mug and, at the time, I was surprised by the price. However, it's not the mug's cost that is important here but what she gets from it, and in particular what she gets from using it every day. The mug represents in physical form a part of her artistic truth, where this is the need for objects to be "simple, beautiful and functional". The mug is all these things and because of this she "enjoys it" and "loves it". My friend is a mother of two, one still a babe in arms, and the mug gives her the opportunity to connect, in a direct way, with a part of herself that for most of the week she has to put to one side. By using the mug a number of times each day she is constantly touching base with her artist self, which is a key part of the true her.

Compare this with the tale of another woman who could be me in the days before cancer. The woman works full-time and works hard for a living. She has a job that pays well but leaves little time for her. At the weekends she goes shopping: it makes her feel good. One of the benefits of working as she does is that she can afford to buy nice things. Today she decides to buy new mugs. There's nothing wrong with the old ones but she's had them a while and would like a change. She wanders around the shops looking at what's on offer. She sees a set of six mugs for £25. It's not a bad price and the mugs would go well with the new kitchen she installed a few months ago. She buys them and when she gets home enjoys arranging them on the shelf.

Do you feel differently about the second story? Does it leave you feeling flatter than the first? This isn't because the first story is real and the second is fiction. It's because the second lacks an emotional core. The first story touches something inside of us and the second one doesn't. Often we spend money to gain pleasure: pleasure we don't get elsewhere. But unless the pleasure we get from an object links into and resonates with the truth of who we are, the pleasure we get from it can only be short lived. And if we're out of touch with our true selves, there is nothing we can buy or own that will fill that aching gap.

Sadly, that's how we live in the West. Our lives have little to do with our true selves and our bodies tell us this, day in and day out. And because we cannot bear to feel this way—stressed, depressed, anxious—we spend money—on houses, cars, clothes, electrical items and holidays—on anything and everything that gives us that 'feel good' feeling. But what we have is never enough. While we can override messages from our bodies for a short while, with the chemicals released by them in response to a shopping fix, these soon fade as the novelty of the purchase fades. Then the background messages of the body come to the fore again and to push down these messages we have to spend more. If you don't believe me try spending money on only essential items for a month or two and see what comes up. Those monks were definitely onto something when they chose austerity as a path!

32

When it comes to taking things inside or projecting them outside most people tend to do both but with a preference for one approach. I wasn't like that. When I say I took everything inside, I mean *everything*. Everything was my fault. It was always my way of being that needed to change, in order to make things better, in order for me to fit in. I was a chameleon, continually adapting myself to my surroundings and because of this I learnt a lot about people and society. Ironically, it was by being so introspective— "thinking too much", my husband would say—that I learnt so much about the external world. And, also ironically, it was as a result of being so completely introspective that I became so completely cut off from the true me.

When you blame others for what happens, although you don't learn from your mistakes and grow, at the same time you don't easily lose touch with who you are. By the act of blaming others you are saying, "I am right and you are wrong", and so hold onto something of yourself. But when you blame yourself for everything, nothing is sacred. Not only do you let go of the bits of you that deserve to be let go of, you also let go of the bits that are fundamentally you and that are essential for your health and well-being. This is what happened to me. I became completely the other me, so much so that I didn't know the true me existed. But the true you cannot be lost completely. It remains within you, hidden by the other you.

To get in touch with the true you, something is needed to remove the other you so that the true you is revealed.

The more stuff you have, i.e. the bigger the other you, the bigger the thing needs to be that can clear it away. I had so much stuff it had to be something as big as cancer. It's as simple as that. But this is not all I need to say here: there are many strands and we're only beginning to see these and how the knot was formed. You also need to understand why the big thing needed to be cancer and not something else, and how I could see cancer for what it was immediately. Luckily these are linked. The answer lies in:

Who is it that I am?
Who is the true me?

I am in love with reality.
I crave the truth.
I delight in moments that make people cringe
and most people try to avoid.

I love when something is revealed.
When the veils of illusion fall down and you see the
cold
hard
glorious
truth.

I love when people argue after a protracted period of
being artificially
and diplomatically
nice.

I love when someone makes a snide remark
and so reveals the truth of who they are.

I love when life stops you in your tracks.
Shattering everything you thought you knew
and everything you believed in.

I love when there's nowhere to hide.
When you don't have a choice
about which way to go.
When the only way
is the way you've been avoiding.

I love when you step outside of yourself
for just long enough
to see things a different way.

Of course, it wasn't always this way. For most of my life
I was the very opposite of this person: the very opposite of
the true me.

33

I need to tell you what the body is. You may guess what I'm about to say from what I've said so far, but I need to be explicit so there's no confusion and to bring us together at this point. Your body is a vessel. It gives the true you a place to be on this earth. It is the means by which you interact with the earth and others on it. Through your body you experience what it means to be alive. By listening to your body and letting it guide, you can find answers to all questions and true joy and happiness — things that cannot be found elsewhere.

Some of you may find this last sentence controversial, perhaps even profane. I'm thinking of those who follow a specific religion and who believe, very strongly, that the answers, joy and happiness are to be found there. To these people I want to say this: "Please bear with me. I'm not out to rubbish your beliefs. I'm simply setting things out in a different way. Please walk with me a little longer and hear what it is I have to say."

Let me begin with the Dalai Lama's words from *Ancient Wisdom, Modern World, Ethics for the New Millennium*. He knows more about this than me and I trust, accept and believe what he says: "...if we consider the world's major religions from the widest perspective...they are all... directed toward helping human beings achieve lasting happiness. And each of them is, in my opinion, capable of facilitating this."

So, if all of us that have religious beliefs are, in the widest sense, heading in the same direction — that of lasting happiness—what of those who choose another path? In the widest sense this applies to other people too. Whatever job, house, hobbies or relationships people have, being happy in them and happy with them is usually one of the main, if not stated, goals. Even people with very base desires—lots of money, for example—usually think that via this route they will find happiness. Above and beyond everything else, happiness is what most people want.

How do you know you're happy?
Or joyous, or fulfilled?
How do you know life is worth living?
Or you're on the right path?

You know because you feel it.
You experience life from that place.
You know, because *your body* tells you so.

Without your body you are nothing.
Because without your body you can feel nothing.
And without this you are lost.

The glory of God.
The power of prayer.
The wonder of enlightenment.
Through the body, we manifest the divine.

34

When you're in touch with the true you—the little bit of you that is God—by definition, the things you say and the things you do are the works of God. Indeed, God can only work through people in this way. (More controversy!)

But it's not the true you that's on my mind right now but the other you. I've had enough of my other me. I've carried her around for nearly 40 years and I'm prepared to do it no longer. I've lived with her silencing me in almost every conversation I had until I got cancer. I've suffered the backlash of her fears and insecurities, seeing them destroy my confidence, my relationships and my ability to be the true me. And, worst of all, I've lived a life where I became progressively smaller. Squashing myself into the shrinking box she made for me until I, in my human form, almost disappeared.

No more!

I've seen who I truly am and I'm not prepared to let that person go—not now, not ever again. This is what I felt the day the doctor told me I had cancer. I had no words to explain it then but this is what I felt. Cancer, with its amazing strength and power, punched through the other me and allowed the light of the true me to shine, reminding me who that person is and flooding me with the wonder of her being. This is why I was euphoric. It had nothing to do with the cancer itself. It was me experiencing the true me: me experiencing the bit of me that is God. And because we are *all* made the same way—all made in the image of

God—we can all feel this way. We simply need to shed the skins of who we've become and see ourselves as we truly are.

Oh, but the shedding of that skin!
How difficult a thing it is to do.

PART FIVE

35

We've not yet reached the point where I can explain how I managed to shed the skin of the other me sufficiently to make the transition from my imaginary world into reality a permanent one. Not that this matters because there are as many words left as I need to tell my story and it will, in the end, be told. However I am growing weary and maybe you are too. There is always a point on a spiritual journey when you feel like giving up. Indeed there are many such points. It's what you do when you get to these that determines your path. At the beginning it's easy to be knocked off course; many things, including people, get in your way. Why is that?

The world out there is not made for spiritual people. It's made for the other you.

To deal with this, I have, to a large extent, cut myself off from it. So that I can hold onto my truth in a world where the truth is just one version of events, I've stopped reading newspapers and stopped watching the news. I read only two magazines on a regular basis and I pick and choose what I watch on television. I watch mainly comedy and reality TV and therein find some hope for the future. That our schedules are awash with reality TV shows must translate into a public interest in reality—and anything real is good. But there's a problem when it's not reality we're seeing but illusion (or delusion) on a grand scale. And in a world made for and populated by the other you, this is what we have.

And every time you interact with it and engage in it, that's what you become—more of the other you.

The closer you get to the true you, the more clearly you see other people—as their true selves or their other selves depending on who they're being. In the past week this has taken a surreal turn for me. When I'm in contact with a person who is clearly being their other self, perhaps fearful or jealous, that person appears as if they have a swarm of something buzzing round them, mainly around the head. This swarm is not tangible in our reality but the person somehow gives the impression of it being there. This is odd to experience but also slightly amusing, and for me that's a good thing. The humour of it opens up the compassionate side of me and I feel warmer towards that person than I would otherwise have done. But this isn't helping—apart from showing what may lie further along your path—and I need to return to my cancer story.

One thing I've not told you is that I was diagnosed on February 14th, Valentine's Day. When I remember this fact it makes me smile. It's not a smile that recollects an amusing event but a smile that acknowledges and marvels at the 'Magician that is Life'. To have a cancer that's all about love and to be diagnosed on Valentine's Day, how magical is that? My cancer came *labelled* with love! And being told in this manner where to look for the next steps of the path, I felt cared for and somehow protected by life. Yes, I had 'been given'—not that I like that phrase—cancer, but at the same time life was saying, "we're here to help you too".

The cancer was not only about the love of my parents but also my love for my ex-husband, my son, my unrequited love and myself. All of these I had to face to set myself free. Looking back I cannot remember what the issues were with people other than my parents—and it's not important to this story. Why can't I remember? Things happened such a long time ago—only three years in elapsed time but so much more than that in terms of how far I've moved and how much I've grown—and I didn't keep a diary or a journal during those times.

When I decided to write this book, that I'd not kept a record of events worried me. But when I shook myself and asked my body, "is this OK?" the answer always came back as "yes". At the time I didn't know why but it makes sense to me now. This book must focus on who I am now and what has made me this way and not on who I was then. It's important that I can go back and talk of the old me but it needs to be from the perspective of here. Any detailed account of the past would draw me back into the person I was then and not, as this book is doing, pull me forward into the person I am to become. I did write some poetry though, in the days after diagnosis, and I'll look back at it to see what I find. Like the fairy tale, there may be much of truth in it.

I'm part way through my review of the poetry but there's something I need to tell you: something that cannot wait. This has been growing for the past week or so. I can trace its almost imperceptible beginning back to the first day I saw my current counsellor. I wrote in the Preface to this book: "I want to experience life as I did with cancer. I want to feel about life the way that I did with cancer". Today, for the first time, life has been that way and I need to take this opportunity to describe it to you, in the moment, as I am living it.

There is a separating out of me from this world, the world of the other you. I am still present in it and part of it, but my energy, and so my experience of it, has shifted out of the banality of the everyday and into the realm of the magical or sacred. This shift has come as a result of being the true me. Not the true me with the other me stuck to it, but the true me alone. I know the other me still exists and will soon reform around me but for the moment who I am is the true me, nothing more and nothing less. My path, as long as I stay on it, will allow me to get here more often and stay for longer each time. Indeed that's all the path is.

36

It's a week later. My son was on holiday from school and I wrote nothing during this time. While this could appear to be a shame—me being stopped in mid-flow after waiting three years to get to this place—in reality it's another example of life stepping in to give me what I need, when I need it. Returning to my computer this morning, I was given the opportunity to reflect on what I'd written from the new space I inhabit. Although a rarity, I deleted some of the text I wrote last week. I did this because I know I wasn't grounded when I wrote it and therefore that it shouldn't be read by you.

I need to stay grounded if I'm to write a book you can relate to. The things I have to say are difficult enough for you to hear, without me flying off into hyperspace and talking to you from there. Staying grounded is difficult though. It's easy to be carried away by the feelings that arise from the true you because they are, quite simply, without equal. So much so that having experienced them once, almost like an addict, you must experience them again—having tasted life as it should be experienced, nothing else will do. I stopped being grounded when I tried to describe what it feels like to experience life as the true you. These feelings are, after all, what made it possible for me to be euphoric following my cancer diagnosis and it's these I've been in pursuit of ever since. It's important, therefore, that I can convey them to you, or at least move you to a place from which you can have some concept of them.

My mind keeps returning to a book I was introduced to in a creative writing course I took in the autumn following my mastectomy. The book is *Ingenious Pain* by Andrew Miller and the extract concerns the performing of a caesarean section, without anaesthetic, on a Mrs Porter in the winter of 1764. "James strips off his coat, opens his bag, selects a knife, examines briefly the rosy skin, then cuts, fast, a vertical incision from belly button to pubic hair. Mrs Porter roars, swings a small white fist with considerable power against his left ear. He laughs, does not look up. He says: 'A good sign, I think. Now hold her still. I have some delicate work here. Jog my knife, Mrs Porter, and you shall bleed to death'."

The tutor asked why the author had chosen to describe the scene in this way, without describing Mrs Porter's feelings. The answer? First, some things are best left to the reader's imagination; second, actions speak louder than words. Nothing Andrew Miller could have said can better the images, feelings and thoughts that come to mind as you consider Mrs Porter—or yourself—being cut, without anaesthetic, from "belly button to pubic hair". Any of us that have experienced pain can imagine the pain involved; yet to describe this pain to another would be impossible. Indeed to attempt a description would be foolhardy, as it would probably result in less of a connection between the reader and the event, rather than more so. However—and this is the good thing—such a description is not needed. The telling of the story is enough to trigger our own memories of pain and for us to extrapolate these to fit what we hear; we do not need to be told in words, when these can only be inadequate.

But how does this relate to me experiencing life as the true me? The same rules apply: some things are best left to the reader's imagination and actions speak louder than words. Experiencing life as the true you is as extreme a thing as being cut by a knife without anaesthetic. And just as it's possible to extrapolate from the pain you've experienced to an idea of extreme pain, so it's possible to extrapolate from the joy and happiness you've felt to this higher level. However, while we can all relate to the feel of the surgeon's knife—because we know enough about it—the same cannot be said of experiencing life as the true you. It's easy with pain. We've all stubbed a toe, fallen as children or cut a knee, and even if we haven't broken limbs, given birth or suffered physical abuse or torture, we know these things can and do happen. They are therefore real to us and their pain is just one imaginative step away. It's not the same with feelings that arise from a spiritual experience—and having come this far I can see this is what I had. And it makes sense, doesn't it?

Woman + cancer = euphoria
Doesn't quite add up

Woman + cancer + an experience of God = euphoria
Now that *does* make sense

But to many people such experiences are not a matter of fact but of belief. And while we tend to believe someone when they tell of experiences that were painful, either physically or emotionally, this is not the case when someone says they've experienced God. That's why we need the second rule: actions speak louder than words. If you want to appreciate the enormity of my experience, look at my actions: refusing a planned mastectomy; giving up my job; selling my house; being happier during cancer than at any other time in my life. These show the scale of my experience and its power.

They show what's possible when
You stop being the other you.

37

This morning, when talking to a friend outside the school gates, I realised something about this book—or rather, I realised something about you. I got a strong sense of who this book is for: people who have no spiritual beliefs to speak of and for whom the sacred is not an experiential reality[14]. I started with the belief that this book is for people with cancer—and it is—but it's not so much this disease that characterises the reader I have in mind but rather the absence of any connectedness with and awareness of the universal positive energy I'm calling God. Why is this book mainly for these people? Because they need it most.

At this point I can imagine you, being one of them, very forcibly closing the book! Telling someone they're in need of something is not the way to win friends and influence people. I'm very aware of this—so much so that I don't want to follow the literary path in the direction it's taking me. So, yet again, this book mirrors life. I find myself in a place I don't want to be, headed somewhere I don't want to go. I could change direction, but that's not the answer. If I restarted the chapter and took a different tack, the spell would be broken and the magic lost.

I must continue in this direction
Because this is the way I *must* go.
The things I fear to say must be said.
There is no other way.

It is the same with life and I feel it strongly now. Just as I
did not want this book to be about God, so it was with my
life. When I emerged from the hospital into the sunshine
of that February morning, I didn't know the reason for the
euphoria or where it would lead me. I knew only that I'd
felt that way before (when I listened to my husband when
he said he wanted to leave), that I'd let the feeling go and
that life without it had been unbearable: a life without life.
Yet here I was being given a second chance to hold onto
this feeling, this time by cancer. And this time I was *not*
going to let it go. No matter what was said or done, no
matter where it took me or what I had to do, I would not
let it go.

It's good to remember this when my life doesn't seem to
be my own. It reminds me this is the path *I* have chosen.
Just because it's not going the way I think it should, doesn't
mean it's the wrong path. I'm simply struggling with it,
that's all. I'm afraid of what it means for me that my life
and this book are about God.

38

It's the next day and I'm in a quandary. I feel I should be writing but at the same time I'm afraid to do so. I've started to question what I'm saying and worrying about loose ends. I wonder if the book holds together. My mind keeps returning to a conversation I had last night with a man I'd just met and will probably never see again.

I was at the pub with a couple of friends. Because it was a lovely evening, the first of the summer, we sat outside. We shared a square table, bench seats on each side, with two university lecturers; they'd been there since lunchtime, enjoying the sun and taking a break from marking. We chatted with them occasionally throughout the evening but the conversation really took off when one of the bar staff removed the folded green and yellow parasol from the centre of the table that had, until that time, obscured each group's view of the other.

We talked of various things until one of my friends mentioned I was writing a book, at which point this and spirituality became the main topic of conversation. My friends and one of the lecturers left early, leaving me with the other, a historian teaching politics. Two things stand out from the conversation, both concern truth.

He said: "There's no such thing as a universal truth."

And I, not in direct response to this but sometime later, said: "The truth cannot be spoken or written, it can only be known." While these statements appear contradictory, we're saying—more or less—the same thing. He might not agree but I'm writing this book!

Why am I telling you this? Because my words provide justification for, or another take on, something I said in the third chapter when I tried to explain why I needed saving by cancer and what from: "That's not going to be easy to explain, is it? Not in a way that gives you a bodily understanding of what I'm talking about. It's no good me telling you how it is, that won't do at all. You need to understand what I am saying not with your head, but with your body. You need to begin to *know*."

This book is written in the way that it is because only in this way can I give you access to truth—your truth. In it I'm recounting what happened to me, what I believe and what this means. This is my story and my truth. Your truth may not be the same as mine—it may well be different—but that doesn't matter. By telling my story and in so doing speaking my truth, I give you access to yours.

Truth is recognised by the body and resonates in it.

39

On my return from hospital on the day of diagnosis, I met the brother of a friend. I asked him in for a cup of tea and when rinsing the teapot I caught it on the tap, breaking part of the spout. I'll take myself back to that moment so I can access the feelings I had at the time...The kitchen sink faces a window. It looks out onto a back yard that is green-tinged from the lichen on the concreted ground. The back of the house is north-facing and gets little sun; even in the height of summer the area outside the window is always in shade. The sink is on the left with a drainer on the right. Both are stainless steel as is the mixer tap that separates the two...

It would have been easy to be angry at breaking the spout; it presented the perfect opportunity to release any energy generated in response to the diagnosis. But it wasn't like that. As the spout hit the tap and I registered the sound of this and the chip falling into the sink, there were no feelings of anger or annoyance. It was, like the cancer, 'just one of those things' and, like the cancer, carried with it a message:

A teapot is a teapot even with a bit of its spout missing. You will be a woman even with the loss of a breast.

I didn't think this way to make a bad situation better and it wasn't a case of positive thinking. I genuinely reacted like this. The teapot is broken, it's showing me something; breast cancer is here for a reason and carries with it a message. I didn't need to convince myself that it was this way because it *was* this way. I knew it to be true.

The brother of a friend didn't know how to respond. His dad had died of cancer, but his silence wasn't to do with that. It wasn't his past experiences that caused him to be silent, but his experience of me. This was the first time I became aware of someone acting this way around me but since then it has happened a number of times. What characterises these moments is the quality of the silence and the look on a person's face. The silence comes from the listening. As when I listened to my husband, the listener puts himself on hold, taking in things only from the outside. The depth of the silence is a direct result of the silencing of inner thoughts — it's not that I can hear people's thoughts but on some level I pick up on them or, as in this case, the absence of them. When it comes to the look that someone has it's slightly quizzical, with an intensity that reflects the nature of the silence rather than any feelings. These moments don't happen when someone is being a know-it-all. Know-it-alls believe exactly that — i.e. they know it all — and thus that there's nothing to be gained from stopping their inner dialogue — not that it would cross their minds to do so — to listen to another person.

The people I encountered when I had cancer fell into two groups: the know-it-alls and the listeners. During cancer the foremost thought in my mind was "I must not let this feeling of euphoria go". I wasn't sure how I'd lost it after my husband left but that didn't matter. I knew if I held onto the feeling this time, everything would be OK. So, how I related to people depended on my experience of them in relation to this feeling. Those who listened and at least tried to embrace how I felt were my confidants and allies; those who thought I was mad were my foes. It was as simple as that. It didn't matter who the people were, the relationship we'd previously had or how I'd felt about them. I allowed this—and only this—to determine our relationship from that point on. In terms of my journey and getting closer to the true me, it was one of the most important things I've done.

Cancer, by its very nature, gave me permission to be that way: permission to be myself. Before cancer I'd been afraid to be me. For one reason and another—fear, insecurity, the need to be liked, the need to fit in—I rarely voiced my true thoughts and allowed factors other than my true feelings to determine the nature of my relationships. I'd got it into my head that I should be able to get along with everyone and developed relationships on that basis. If the relationship wasn't going well, I took it that *I* was doing something wrong and that *I* needed to change and adapt. It's that way of thinking that, in part, let the know-it-alls get to me when my husband left.

40

I'm drawn to tell you of the ending of a friendship in the run up to cancer. It feels right to tell this story but I'm also aware that I may be opening old wounds for the person involved. She took the ending of the friendship badly and for the ham-fisted way in which I dealt with it, I'm sorry. I'm also sorry that I allowed the friendship to develop as it did for it's this that caused the problems for me.

I'll start by sharing the moment I realised the friendship had to end. I was on the way home after dropping my son at nursery; walking down a hill, alongside a main road, on the outskirts of the city—not the suburbs, closer in than that. I'm struck by how clear the picture is, not so much the road itself—I walked that four times every weekday—but my sense of being there, in that moment, in that space.

A minute or so after leaving the nursery I started to feel odd. There were no specific physical sensations—no pain, no dizziness, no sickness—but something wasn't right. Being me I asked, "what's wrong?" and as I walked down the road an image began to form. It started as a feeling that energy was draining out of me, then I saw a picture of myself as a cartoon character shot full of holes. Accompanying this was an awareness that my relationship with my friend was affecting me in this way—it was draining me—and given this I had to end it. So that's what I did, with a letter, a day or so before Christmas. The coward's way out and appalling timing but at the time I could do nothing else.

To explain why things had to be this way I need to flip forward to cancer then jump back again. It's hard for me to say the things I have to say though, because they involve another person. However I'm only discussing this person in terms of her impact on me—it's my story, so I do not need her permission—and, as I've said, it was me allowing the friendship to develop as it did that caused the problems.

People are the way they are; we cannot change them. Instead of focusing on what we believe to be wrong with someone, we need to concentrate on our behaviour given the actions of this person. In this way our choices become clear. There are many reasons why people do not listen. Sometimes being a know-it-all is simply a matter of seeing only how you feel and not being aware of the feelings of others.

A week after my diagnosis I bumped into an old school friend; we sat next to each other when we were eleven. She had seen my 'unceremoniously dumped' friend the day before in the supermarket, distraught and crying in the aisles because I had cancer. I'd known before then that it was right for me to end the friendship but this confirmed it. Because of the nature of my friend and the nature of our relationship, it would have been difficult for me to hold onto my truth around her.

I see the cartoon image of me shot full of holes as the beginning of my body's conversation concerning cancer. Although this predated the lump it was only by a matter of weeks and I believe the cancer was already in my body at this time. Perhaps—but this is wishful thinking: what a great story!—this image was my body's response to the growth of the first cancerous cell.

The relationship with my friend was not so different from my other friendships in that I withheld a part of myself, however in this relationship it was at its most extreme. By the end of the friendship I was withholding virtually all of myself and it is this (and nothing else) that meant the friendship had to end. It is because I wanted to be this person's friend that I started withholding myself and because I wanted to make the friendship work that it lasted so long—about seven years. By the time I realised what harm it was doing to me to withhold myself to such a large extent, it was too late to do anything other than I did, i.e. end the friendship. Too much had happened and too many things had been left unsaid.

That my body chose to speak to me about cancer by highlighting this relationship shows the immense wisdom of the body. Above and beyond anything else, it is the withholding of myself that I have had to give up, to ensure that the move to the true me has been a permanent one.

PART SIX

41

For a long time I struggled with the idea of a mastectomy. This wasn't because I feared the operation would destroy my femininity—remember the teapot—but because I wasn't convinced it was a necessary step. Looking at it from here, I can see my struggles were little more than a delaying tactic. I wasn't trying to avoid the operation—although that's how it appeared to me and everyone else—instead I was putting it off until I was ready to go forward with it, without the risk of falling back into old ways.

None of this was clear at the time. Then I had only feelings that I knew I had to follow but that didn't make sense from an intellectual perspective. This is the main reason people had difficulty with me. What I was saying didn't make sense, but how could it make sense when I didn't understand my feelings? How I acted didn't make sense either, but how could I have acted in a rational way when rationality had nothing to do with it?

There are tears in my eyes now, some on my cheeks and some in my lap. If I'd not hung onto my truth during those eleven weeks between the cancer diagnosis and the mastectomy, I would now be lost. The bit of me that is me and nothing else, the part that defines 'Lesley' and gives me access to love, joy and happiness unlike any other, would be buried beneath the other me, unable to breathe, to stretch and to grow.

What I'm aware of in writing these words is not only how important it was for me to hang onto my truth, but also how amazing it is that I managed it. My mum and dad, my doctors and most of my friends thought I was mad and risking my life by delaying the operation, yet I knew—without being able to express it and without knowing why—that it was, in fact, the other way round. If I'd been weaker, if I'd listened to others, if I'd let any one of the know-it-alls in, I'd be back in that dark, depressing and deathly space that was the time before cancer. And if cancer hadn't got me out of it, could anything have done?

I need to talk about the knowing, the one that kept me on track. I'll start by taking you back to my words from Chapter 2: "The thing about knowing is that's what it is: *knowing.* You don't know why you know, or how you know, you just know. You know it in your body—in that place between your belly button and your heart...When you *know*, you don't know anything apart from the fact that you know."

If there are words that have an effect on me unlike any others, it is these: "I've got a feeling I should do something but I don't know why." Upon hearing them my body straightens slightly and tenses and I move a little closer to the person, head edging forward. My pupils dilate and there is a look of excitement in my eyes—I must be a little scary!—and what I say comes out of my body with such energy, power and conviction: "Then you must do it! Above and beyond anything else, this is what you must do!"

But most people are not like me when it comes to decision-making—not when it comes to big decisions and certainly not life-and-death ones. While it's OK to follow feelings in relation to small things that 'don't really matter', for important decisions such as where to live, what job to do and whether to listen to the advice of doctors, people tend to follow their rational side. But not always. People often choose a house based mainly on a feeling. While there will be criteria to meet such as general location, number of bedrooms and size of garden, many people opt for the property that feels right: "I knew this was the one as soon as I walked through the door."

This is the *knowing* I talk about and it's possible to enhance and develop it so that you can apply it to every aspect of your life. But to do this you need to listen to it and follow it without exception, wherever and whenever it appears, and this is not easy because, houses aside, our knowing often takes us in a different direction from our rational side. But that's where my story can help. By showing what I've gained from trusting my knowing—and what I appeared to be risking—I'm opening your eyes to the possibility of trusting yours too.

Between the cancer diagnosis and the mastectomy my knowing was little more than that. I didn't understand it and I couldn't express it in any way other than to say, "I must do this." But it wasn't as simple as that. If I was in the same position now, having experienced what I've experienced and knowing what I know, I wouldn't try to explain it to most people. But back then I was a different person and at times a scared and confused one and because of that, and because I was trying to make sense of my feelings, I did discuss it. But, as I've said before, only with those who were prepared to listen and hold back their views.

Following my knowing was particularly hard for my mum and dad. They thought me wrong to act as I did—and they probably still feel that way; our differences were so extreme we've not resolved them. We've not talked about what happened, reconciled our differences and moved on; instead we've pushed it under the carpet, all glad that the period of disagreement is over. We've moved on, but only to the extent that we can move on given that the issue, while buried, is still alive.

It's interesting to acknowledge this because that's how most of us deal with issues in our lives: we don't resolve them. Instead we wait until they're no longer current, then forget about them. It's this approach to life, along with others, that creates, so quickly and effectively, the other you. By saying this, I'm admitting to the creation and maintenance of a part of the other me, which has arisen from me not talking to my parents about how I behaved during cancer. Hurrah! I'm fallible! Just like you. And although I've said that in a humorous way (that was the intention), it's important that you do see me in this way, i.e. just like you. To believe we are different is illusion. Everything I have done, you are capable of doing also. All that stops you is the other you.

This is why cancer is an amazing and incredible thing to have and welcome into your life. It is a colossus—a thing of gigantic power and influence—and because of that it's able to do what you are unable to do for yourself, i.e. to contain and silence, if only for a little while, the all-powerful and insidious other you. Think about it for a moment. What occupied your mind and/or worried you before you had cancer? What happened to those things when cancer came along? My guess is they disappeared, albeit, for some of you, not for long.

This is what cancer is for.
This is its purpose.
This is its power.

And if enough of the other you can be shut down, what you see and get access to is the true you.

42

In the days before cancer my life was so full. One of the things I've not talked about until now is the impact of cancer on my working life. I didn't stop working when I had cancer but one thing I did do—something that before cancer had seemed impossible—was to stop being a workaholic. Yet with cancer I did it overnight.

It was hard being a single parent and running my own business, especially when my son was so small—eighteen-months when my husband left and four-and-a-little-bit when I was diagnosed. I worked in the morning when my son was at nursery and again in the evening when he'd gone to bed. And in the early days I had even less child-free time to work. When my husband left I set up my business, using the two hours in the afternoons when my son slept. About a year or so later my ex had him two days a week and I worked then. However, this became untenable for both of us—my ex needing time to work himself and me needing time across the whole week—so nursery it was, mornings only; I could not bear my son to attend for the whole day.

I didn't know I was a workaholic. I thought my workaholism—not that I called it that—was a product of my circumstances and that it had to be that way. I didn't realise I had a choice—I needed cancer to show me that—nor did I see or understand what lay beneath. Workaholism was one of the ways—one of the many ways—I held together the world of the other me.

There are as many expressions of the other you as there are people, and as many expressions of the truth. However, people's other-you behaviour falls into categories that can be identified and defined. Workaholism, alcoholism and drug addiction are three such categories but there are many, many more. Some are more extreme, such as physical and sexual abuse, but many others are more moderate in nature. They are commonplace and widely accepted in our society; considered reasonable, even. What I have in mind are the Seven Deadly Sins. In case you don't know what they are, or need to be reminded, here's a description.

The Seven Deadly Sins are transgressions that are fatal to spiritual progress: "*Pride* is excessive belief in one's own abilities, that interferes with the individual's recognition of the grace of God. It has been called the sin from which all others arise. Pride is also known as vanity. *Envy* is the desire for others' traits, status, abilities or situation. *Gluttony* is an inordinate desire to consume more than one requires. *Lust* is an inordinate craving for the pleasures of the body. *Anger* is manifested in the individual who spurns love and opts instead for fury. It is also known as wrath. *Greed* is the desire for material wealth or gain, ignoring the realm of the spiritual. It is also called avarice or covetousness. *Sloth* is the avoidance of physical or spiritual work."[15]

When I revisited these sins two things struck me. Firstly, how they have been misrepresented and secondly, how Western society has embraced them as qualities to be aimed for, rather than avoided! In the descriptions of both gluttony and lust the word "inordinate" is used; it means, "unrestrained: excessive: immoderate" (Chambers)—so there's nothing wrong with lust (yippee!) as long as it's not inordinate. And pride and greed are defined, not in relation to the individual, but in terms of their impact on spiritual progress, or the recognition of God. But this message has been lost and, instead, the Seven Deadly Sins have been sharpened. We have been led to believe that within a spiritual life, all lust, all pride, all greed is wrong. Thus a spiritual life has moved out of reach of the vast majority of people and we have, instead, a society that ignores the spiritual in favour of the material and scientific. And the result? A society hell bent (excuse the pun) on manifesting the Seven Deadly Sins.

We're told to look more attractive and younger, to aim for higher paid jobs and corporate responsibility. Rather than be content with what we have, we strive for more of everything. Ours is a society built on greed. True, a spiritual path is not an easy one. But once established on it any other path becomes — through choice — unacceptable. And yet it's not the difficulties we should be focusing on but the rewards. And the rewards that are to be gained in this lifetime and not just the next.

43

The decision not to have the planned mastectomy was the turning point and yet, in this story, we have not quite reached it. We are at the day before, the day spent with one of my friends. It was late April and we went to Wells, on the North Norfolk coast; our intention, to spend time on the beach in touch with nature and in solitude. In hindsight this was a good choice, solitude being the chosen path of many a saint and monk across the years. It was a truly fabulous day; a clear, crisp blue sky typical of spring, with the warmth of a summer sun. My friend read a book while I wandered along the beach in search of...In search of what exactly? A sign to show me the way.

I lay in the dunes, staring at the sky, watching the clouds. Thinking of that time has brought back to me a shape I saw there, something I'd forgotten. And yet it is this that preceded the sign, although it wasn't a sign telling me where I should go, but marking out where I'd been. Lying on the beach I was in another place. Pushed out of the world of the other me by the size of the decision I had to make, and drawn into another world—the world of the magical or sacred—via the energy of nature and my longing for my truth. The clouds took on the shape of a pair of breasts—certainly specific enough to grab my attention—and above my head buzzed a bee. Busy, busy, busy. Busy, busy, busy. Busy, busy, busy. It was clear. Part of what had brought me to cancer was the busyness of my life in the years before.

It wasn't simply a case of being a workaholic. There were other things I'd crammed into my life to avoid facing the truth, not that I knew I was doing this or what the truth was. Between my husband leaving and my body giving me cancer, I became involved in local politics, a local charity and a community group. These didn't run concurrently, instead one followed the other, overlapping slightly, always giving me something to do—something to eat up my time. The eating up of time wasn't all I got from these organisations; they gave me something too. But while this seemed to be what I wanted, and at the time enough, it never resonated with the truth of who I am as deeply as does my current path and the writing of this book.

It's not a completely dark picture I should be painting though. I did get satisfaction from these organisations and, in swapping one for another, I was, each time, stepping closer to my path and my truth. The community group was very close to my heart and had life not stepped in to prevent my involvement, I'd have continued with it. My ex-husband had been looking after our son on the evenings the group met, but after breaking up with his then partner (just before I found the first lump) he moved to another city and was unable to continue. Without regular childcare I felt unable to carry on with the group—I was its Chair— and so, with great sadness, I resigned.

But that is where life has been particularly generous to me—in giving me what I need when I need it—although, because of the nature of the gifts, that's not how most people see it. I would not have given up my role in the community group without being pushed. Just like my artist friend's mug, the group allowed me to touch base with a key part of the true me; indeed, only by being a member of this group did I become aware this part of me existed. But I needed to break away from the group to move forward to where I am now and that is where my ex-husband's move came in. Life, via him, forced my hand, and I am grateful to it.

The timing of his previous move was important for me also. He'd left only three months after I'd given up my full-time, well-paid job of seven years to be a full-time mum supported by him. Some considered him a bastard for doing this but I knew that, had he left before I'd given up my job, I wouldn't have had the courage to do it. And leaving my job was definitely something I needed to do. Life always gives you what you need to thrive and to grow—to become strongly and more fully the true you. But because what you want is often different from this—to stay firmly and securely the other you—what life gives you is often misinterpreted. Life's gifts are, therefore, seen as upsets and tragedies and we, the recipients of universal love, are seen as merely the victims of circumstance.

But after that bit of profundity—makes a change from profanity!—I'll return to the day before my proposed mastectomy. As I look back, my body takes on the feeling of that time and I'm struck by the heaviness of it. All of my weight is concentrated in the centre of my body, towards my heart chakra and my solar plexus, and that area is exerting a strong pull on the rest of me, drawing me into this point. It is from here that the *knowing* comes and maybe that is what was happening. I was being pulled into my knowing which is, after all, what I was asking for.

From the beach we made our way to the Shrine of Our Lady of Walsingham, for many centuries a place of pilgrimage. My friend and I split up, preferring to wander around the church and grounds separately—or maybe she was giving me the space and time I needed on my own. I remember writing a request for prayer: slips of paper are provided to write the names of people for whom you want the nuns to pray. I wrote my name on one and on another two, the names of my parents. I remember watching a service in one of the side chapels. I stood at the back and felt not quite part of it; unable to receive communion because I have not been confirmed. I remember taking a sip of holy water from a white plastic cup.

Later, I sat in the chapel where people light candles in return for a small fee. I don't know how long I sat there or how many words passed through my mind. All I remember is what happened as one word entered my consciousness. It was a bright day, but with clouds in the sky. It was gloomy in the centre of the building and, with the candles burning, it seemed more like evening than the height of day. A cloud must have completed its path across the sun, so allowing the sun's rays to shine through the windows of the church, flooding the chapel with light. For me, sitting in the chapel, this happened in the blink of an eye. One moment I was in semi-darkness, the next in the brightest of lights. And the word that accompanied this illumination?

Faith.

It's not possible to convey what that moment meant, not in a way that can hold on to its magic. I think I shared it with my friend on the way home, but even then my attempts at explanation somehow detracted from the event rather than added to it. It's OK for me to write about what happened—and I need to because it's an important part of the story—but it's for you to put yourself in my place and to see, or perhaps feel, your way forward with it. What I can say is that this moment did not change everything— it wasn't one of those. But somehow the brightness and warmth of the sunshine carried the experience of faith, or rather an appreciation of it, deep into my body.

44

The next day I woke early. The operation was planned for nine and I had to be there by seven, but I didn't know what to do. I remember sitting in my dressing gown on the floor by the 'phone, not knowing—and it's important that you understand this, because although the knowing was there at times, sometimes I didn't know at all. In a way these times of not knowing are the most important ones. It's easy to follow your knowing when you're in touch with it and clear about it—anyone can do that—but to stay on the path when you don't know, that's hard. In those times faith is important—faith in something bigger than you and an innate trust in yourself, i.e. a belief that you'll do the right thing—but beyond that, you need an understanding that it's OK not to know.

We cannot know all the time. It would be nice but it's not realistic. Life demands that we move forward into the unknown and that there are, by definition, times of not knowing. However society is built around the illusion of moving forward into the known and we fail to see this. Much of our time in the West is spent developing a secure future, but within the boundaries and restrictions of the world of the other you there can be no such thing. Why? Because the true you will always take steps to shatter illusion and reveal truth. Or, as the other you sees it, the true you will always upset things.

Why didn't I have the planned mastectomy? Because I wasn't ready. In the end that's all it came down to. It wasn't a strong feeling of not being ready—it wasn't a knowing—

and at the time and looking back at it now, it feels as if it could have gone either way, i.e. that I could have opted for the operation as easily as I opted out of it. But is that true? I wonder. Is that true? I think not. But what this questioning has drawn my attention to, is how subtle a thing the turning point was. It was the turning point, I have no doubt about that, because after it the knowing took on a new form. It had substance. It had words. But the turning point itself, that was a different thing. It could so easily be missed or dismissed (as shown by my doubts about it), or mistaken for something else; there is a sense that it was just chance that sent me the way of no operation and not the other. But reading back over this section the word that seems appropriate is fate. I have a sense that it was fate that sent me the way of no operation.

Yes. That is what it was: fate.
Heavily disguised as other things.
But that is what it was.

45

In the days that followed me cancelling the planned mastectomy, two realisations told me I'd made the right choice and was headed in the right direction. I was lying in the bath, thinking I guess, when what came to mind completely out of the blue was, "some things are more important than life and death", and with it a knowing that this was true. It's hard to grasp, isn't it? But that's the way it is. It harks back to days of old where purity, honour and virtue—not of the body but of the soul—were tenets to be upheld, as opposed to today's goals of security and wealth.

It cannot be taught.
Maybe it can be learnt.
It cannot be understood.
It can only be known.
And like the wisdom of this book
It must grow in you.
Born of your truth and experience.

What this realisation gave me was a glimpse of the wonders to come. Imagine walking down a long, dark corridor and unexpectedly coming across a stained-glass window that had been hidden from view. Light shines into the corridor through the window and your path, for the first time, can be seen. You know you're on the right path and are excited by what you see. Knowing that some things are more important that life and death, especially when you have a life-threatening disease, is a powerful thing indeed.

The second realisation followed days later. Walking down the road, headed for the shops at the bottom of the hill, "you need to be close to the edge", popped into my head and with it an appreciation of why I'd refused the planned mastectomy. Since Chapter 29 I've been trying to tell you how I ensured that the transition from my imaginary world into reality was a permanent one. We are nearly at the point where this can be told. The key to my escape was to live close to the edge, and what better way to do that than to refuse a mastectomy with a grade III cancer in my breast, growing at the rate of pea to plum to tangerine.

I need to say something about my physical relationship to the lump and now is the time to do so. Hard as it was for anyone to accept, the lump was my friend. It was because of the lump that I found myself and without it I was afraid I'd be lost. I obtained great comfort from sitting with the lump, cradling it in my hand. As I held onto the lump, so I held onto my truth. So it was, therefore, the cancer I had difficulty letting go of. Yes, people at the time did think I was mad. But now that you have come this far you're beginning to understand, aren't you?

I'm not sure when it was in the month between the planned and the actual mastectomy that I went to speak to my mum and dad. I think it was, and let's say it was, somewhere in the middle. It was another one of those fate things—or rather, it may not be fate, this thing I have touched upon and am about to discuss further, but people use this term and you, therefore, may know it by that name. Knowing that some things are more important than life and death gave me, not only an awareness of my path, but also a knowing that this *was* my path. And what this consideration of fate has given me is the awareness that this path has *always* been my path—I simply needed to find it, that's all. And this is how it has to be for there is only one true you and, therefore, only one true path to follow.

The confusion comes from the world you are born into—the world of the other you. Born in this form, of this time, of your parents and into the land of your birth, the experiences you have shape and define your humanity, so giving birth to the other you. As the other you gathers strength and grows so, if you are not careful or fortunate, the true you goes underground and lays hidden. But the world of the other you is not real—it is not permanent— and within you the true you is inviolate. Both eternal and divine, it will make itself known. The truth will be spoken. But for this to be the case—for the true you to be born again, as the Christians say—the other you must fade and die. It is possible, in this time and in this place, for the true you to manifest itself within your earthly body—but only if the other you relinquishes its hold. If it does not, or if it is that time, for the true you to be born again, your earthly body must die.

But there is no defeat in death
Unless we make it so.

46

I've noticed how short the chapters are and how succinct my writing is. I've wondered if I'm rushing to the end, and I may be, but there is another reason for the way things are. Yet again this book mirrors life. Once the way has been cleared—when, in order to move forward, all that needs to be done (or said) has been done (and said)—progress is rapid. When you are on your path—the path of the true you—life opens up for you. What you need is given.

When diagnosed with cancer I was seeing a counsellor. This had nothing to do with the cancer (my first meeting pre-dated the lump), but it was helpful to be seeing her during this time as it gave me someone independent to talk to—someone without an agenda. However much a person wants to support you through an illness such as cancer, if she has something invested in you, via a friendship or other relationship, it's hard for her to put her own wants and needs to one side and think only of you. What's even harder, is for her to put aside her beliefs about the way things are and see things from a different perspective. A person's desire for you to live is partly motivated by the thought of what she would lose by your death. However, this want also stems from a widely held belief that death is to be avoided at all costs. Yet such beliefs are—almost without exception, I'd say—held by those who have no concept of what death really is, and what the real cost is of avoiding it.

I had a conversation with two men in the park the other day—the same park that gave me the woman and her dog. They were Muslims and unlike most conversations I have in the park this one concerned religion, spirituality and God or Allah. I was not aware of the similarities between Islam and Christianity, in particular a belief in life after death, and when sharing views on this topic I found myself saying, for the first time, something I've since realised is important to me and to this story. It concerns how we see life after death, or rather the perspective from which we see it.

We see life after death from here — the world of the other you — and so we see it in those terms. We see ourselves in this body, reunited with friends and family, happy ever after and living out eternity in this way. I can think of nothing worse than for life after death to be like this; for me to be confined within the boundaries of my human form and thus subject to, and imprisoned by, its many limitations. The true you is boundless and timeless, both eternal and infinite.

We're mistaken when we look at life after death from the perspective of the other you; instead we should be viewing life on earth through the eyes of the true you. Only then does life make sense. Only then does it have purpose and meaning. I guess you want me to tell you what the purpose and the meaning is. Sorry, life doesn't work that way. It's for you to discover the true you. It's for you to walk that path. All I can do is draw your attention to it. Whether you choose this or the path of the other you is up to you. Your fate lies in your hands.

But back to my counselling sessions at the time of 'shall I or shan't I have a mastectomy?' During a session after the planned mastectomy, I realised I had to talk to my mum and dad. I can't remember the conversation that lead to this realisation or anything that was said that day. All I know is that it became obvious to me that I had to speak to my parents and luck, or rather life, had it that I was given both the space and the means to do so the very next day. So I had both the desire and the opportunity to talk to my parents. But what finally gave me the strength and courage to do it? The cancer—of course! But because *even that* wasn't big enough to break me out of my imaginary world, what really tipped the balance was cancelling the planned mastectomy: me walking close to the edge.

I'm a strong person—I guess you can see that—but before cancer I used my strength in completely the wrong way. I thought I was using it for my benefit—and I was, but for the benefit of the other me. The flip side was that my strength was also being used against me—against the true me. Until I cancelled the mastectomy I'd avoided speaking my truth to my mum and dad. I had, long before, convinced myself that I didn't need to do so. I believed—the other me believed—I could carry on happily without it. But when I walked close to the edge and as a result could see what I needed to do, the fact that I'd risked my life to get there meant that I *had* to go forward—I no longer had a choice about it. This is where people got me wrong. They thought I was wrong to refuse the planned mastectomy because I was risking my life—but such an action only looks wrong from the world of the other you. I needed to risk my life— the life of the other me—because only in this way could I up the stakes sufficiently to force my hand.

Death is stronger than the other you.
Faced with it, the other me could not possibly win.

47

Although talking to my mum and dad changed everything, I'm not sure anymore what was said. I have a general idea about it, and I'll share this with you in a minute, but it's more important for me to tell you why my memory is not clear: the details are not important and too much detail in this story would be a bad thing. The more you know of the detail of my life, the more distinct I become. However, the picture formed in your mind would be of the other and not the true me. You need to know something of this person to understand who I was and where I came from, but too much information about her and I run the risk of you relating to her and not to me. And there would be no benefit in that. Only the other you can relate to the other me and it is not to this person I wish to speak.

In terms of this story all you need to know is that I said to my parents what I needed to say in order to escape from the world of the other me, but that I have already said and so you must need a little more. It happened then, and I've seen it since, that the speaking of a truth as it is understood by one person changes the nature of reality. Or to be exact, because most of the time we live in a world of illusion, the speaking of a truth allows that illusion to alter. I'm aware that I'm talking of a spoken truth and yet previously I've said, "the truth cannot be written or spoken, it can only be known". I therefore need to distinguish between truth in the world of reality and truth in the world of illusion (i.e. truth as expressed by the true you and truth as expressed by the other you), for these are not the same at all. In both worlds truth is a powerful thing—perhaps the most powerful thing there is—and it is perhaps because of this, and the fact that it is freely and equally available to all, that the truth has become so devalued in the world of the other you.

For every action taken there is a price to pay. Breaking this down into its most basic terms either an action will strengthen and uphold the illusory world or it will weaken and destroy it. It is often as a result of withholding truth that the illusory world is perpetuated. That my parents didn't love me was not true, but in my world—the world of the other me—I believed this and therefore it was true to me. I don't know why the speaking of this 'imagined truth' made a difference, but that is surely what it did. This was the thing I gave myself time to do when I cancelled the operation. This was the thing I needed to do to make sure I didn't slip back into the person I was before cancer. Walking forward into the unknown I didn't know what I was doing or why, I knew only that I had to face whatever came up and do whatever was required.

This is why cancer was such an amazing time for me and part of what I've been trying to recreate ever since: the ability to go forward in life, regardless of the fear and the perceived consequences. Cancer gives you that, and for this reason, it truly is a magical thing. We see cancer as death wrapped up in another name, yet viewed in a different way it is the very opposite of this—the means by which to live.

All that stops you is you: the other you.
All you need to make you happy is you: the true you.

Cancer separates one from the other as nothing else can (save for other life threatening diseases) and if you can find it within yourself to do so, it is something to be thankful for and to cherish. But cancer is not a gift to be held on to and as soon as it has worked its magic, it's time to let it go.

PART SEVEN

48

Some of you will not want me to go forward—those who fear cancer has not yet worked its magic on them. To these people I need to say this: "it is safe for me, and for you, to carry on". There are parts of the other you that are not yet ready to let go, parts that are not yet ready to die. Their desire to hold on to you manifests itself in your emotions and what you feel is fear. But this fear is not real. Fear cannot harm you. It is only your reaction to fear that has power. If cancer is to be for you what it was for me, it *will* be it. Have no fear of that. And for all of you I have a story, another fairy tale.

Once there was a city, a vast city spanning many counties and districts. The inhabitants of the city were happy with their lot and grateful to the powers that be for the privileges they enjoyed. The city was known across the land as the City of Dreams. Everyone knew of its riches and many wished to live there, but the gates of the city were closed to newcomers and had been for some time. No one was allowed in or out of the city but the latter was of no consequence, for no one wished to leave.

One day a cloud blew over the city. There had been clouds before and so there was nothing unusual in that. But this cloud was different because once it had blown across the city walls, it stayed. It was not always in the same area above the city, it drifted from place to place, but it never left the walls of the city, not once in all the time it was there.

It was a while before the people noticed the cloud, it being one of many, but there was something different about this cloud that, in the end, made people notice it. It never changed or grew, it was always the same and it had a very distinct shape. There is no point me describing the shape to you because the cloud, like the city, is long gone. All I need say is that the cloud was different enough that people remembered it and on seeing it again, sometime later, they were surprised.

It started with one or two people mentioning the cloud in passing—you know what it's like, people like to talk about the weather—and as people shared their experience of the cloud so word of the cloud grew. More and more people saw it and noticed it and saw it and noticed it again when it returned to their district.

I'm not sure how long it was before the cloud began to change, but thinking about it, it must have been long enough for everyone to see and notice the cloud at least twice. Long enough for everyone to become aware of it and to comment on its never-changing nature. And maybe it is because the cloud heard everybody say, "it's always the same", that it decided it was time to change.

The cloud started by changing colour—just a little bit, mind you. So little, in fact, that the change was indistinguishable to the naked eye. Most people did not notice the change but there was a man who had been studying the cloud for some time, using the best-available scientific instruments, and he noticed the change straight away. But no one was much interested in what he had to say. I mean, a little change that no one can see, that's not worth anybody's attention, is it?

Not getting the reaction it expected, the cloud tried a little harder to be different and at its very centre created a shining star. The cloud did not know how it had managed to do this but was happy to have done so. It was certain that, now it had changed in this way, the people would notice it was different. Some people spotted the star immediately and within the space of a year it had been seen by everyone in the city. However, most of them dismissed it as something caught up in the cloud—they thought it must be a shiny weather balloon, or something similar, that gave the cloud its sparkle. The children believed otherwise—that somehow the cloud had drawn down one of the stars from the night sky and had given it a place to live, both night and day—but though the adults humoured them, none believed this to be true.

The cloud was surprised by the reaction of the people and did not know what to do. It had worked hard to create the star and was not sure it would be able to change again but wanting the people to see it in a different way, this it tried to do. It was hard for the cloud to change into something new, but this time it surpassed itself and transformed into a bird—the most beautiful bird you have ever seen.

The people did not notice the disappearance of the cloud—it had never been consistently in their lives, always drifting in and out of it—but the bird! That, people did see. And once they'd seen it, what they wanted more than anything was to see it again. It was as if the bird had magical powers and that just the sight of it could make your problems disappear and happiness come your way. But now that the cloud had become the bird, the people were not happy for it to live as it had done, drifting from place to place. This gave them no guarantee of when they would see the bird and thus when they would feel happy. They were also afraid that the bird would leave the city and never return again.

Every day the newspapers gave a report of where the bird had been sighted and where it was expected next. They were never accurate with their predictions but still they caused chaos. Such was the people's desire to see the bird that they would turn up where the bird was expected to be, hoping to catch sight of it. This caused major problems, with many people moving through the city and some skipping work just to see the bird. So bad did these problems become that the rulers of the city decided they must take action. They decided that the easiest thing would be to catch the bird and cage it, giving people turns in access to it. Some people objected, of course, to the capture of the bird, but they were easily outnumbered by the others.

However hard the rulers tried they were unable to catch the bird. It never seemed to come down to earth, it never ate and it never rested. Of course, had they known that the bird was in fact the cloud in a different form this would have made sense, but the people had forgotten about the cloud following the bird's arrival and did not notice it was gone. A proclamation was issued, making it the duty of every citizen to report on the bird's location and to catch it if they could. Special forms were devised for the reporting and were issued to each household. Each family was also required to come up with a plan to catch the bird and to submit this, in writing, to the rulers, once a month.

For a while the people were happy to do this and engaged in their task willingly. But after a while they got tired and bored. The city, as I have said, was a vast one and spanned many counties and districts. It was only rarely that people saw the bird and being made to look out for it all the time somehow took away the enjoyment of it. And although in the beginning it was good to think that you may be the one who came up with the idea that captured the bird, because nothing anyone came up with came even close to working, in the end people got bored with that too and the ideas dried up.

Somehow, people's relationship to the bird changed too. Whereas the sight of it had once filled their hearts with joy, now when they saw it they began to begrudge it slightly, seeing it as a reminder of their failings. And although this took a long, long time, in the end they began to ignore the bird when it visited their district. This started as a deliberate ignoring where they would catch sight of it from the corner of their eye and look away, pretending to see something else. But ended up as a belief that the bird did not, in fact, exist. They did not see it, so it was not there. It was not there, so it did not exist.

The rule of the land still stated that sightings of the bird were to be reported and plans for its capture were to be made, but because people had forgotten about the bird, these laws too were forgotten. After a while the bird even forgot itself. Of course the bird knew it existed and was happy to be a bird—flying where it wanted, when it wanted to—but it forgot that it had once been a cloud; a different thing altogether. So the people forgot the bird and the bird forgot the cloud, but the cloud did not forget the people and that is why it never left the city.

49

Part of this book's power comes from the immediacy of the writing. From the bubbling up of ideas (truths) from whoever is in charge at the time—mostly the true me but sometimes the other one creeps in.

It is not enough that my story is told; you must live it with me for the short while we are together.

Today I'm struggling with my transition from the other to the true me. However much I want to move away from her, I'm finding it hard to let go of the other Lesley. This is, as suggested by my counsellor yesterday, because she has served me well and thus I need to honour her in her passing.

Until this point in time—and thus this point in the book—I have spoken harshly or unkindly about the other me. I was this way because this is how I needed to be to escape her control; she needed to be the enemy so that I could move away from her. But having reached a place where the true me is strong and well established within my body, I am able to look at the other me sympathetically and, dare I say it, with love.

There is nothing intrinsically wrong with the other me. Unlike the other you of some people she has no very dark side, but she is wrong for me. She developed to protect me when I was growing up. However, now she cages and constricts me and I cannot breathe when I am inside her. I have outgrown her, and she must go.

For three years letting go of the other me has been the focus of my life. Whatever I have been called upon to do, I have done, including refusing a mastectomy, giving up my job and selling my house. Apart from what is needed to look after my son and to function on a day-to-day basis as a human being, all of my energies are devoted to the uncovering of the true me and the eradication of the other one. This is my life: I want no other. And yet today the letting go of her brings not the expected joy, but sorrow.

Some time has passed since I wrote the last sentence and I still do not know what it is I'm crying for. I cannot see what it is about the loss of her that saddens me so. Although I get glimpses of the truth these are too fleeting to grasp and to understand, and most of the time I see nothing. It has something to do with her humanness, of that I am sure, but more than this I do not know. And the more I want to see the meaning in all this, the less I know. Reading back over this chapter I can see the problem. I have shifted from being with the sorrow to trying to work out what it is—and this is not the same thing at all. Realisation and understanding come out of the experience of being human, not from the workings of the brain.

It is not her who is sad—this other me—but me who is sad for her. This is not a sadness at her passing, but a sadness for the very nature of her. Possible now because I am more distant from her and thus able to see her for what she is. As she is no longer my master, I am able to view her with compassion. At every stage she did what she thought was best for me. Her aim was to protect me and keep me safe from harm. And in this way she is the same as every other you: whatever means are chosen, protection and safety are always the goals.

With this understanding my view of her has changed

slightly. She is still someone to escape from, but my respect and thanks are also required. She is a guardian who has not recognised that her child has grown and no longer needs the same level of care and attention. I must therefore fight her to get away but not allow myself to forget her past good deeds. And because I am not—none of us ever are—fully grown, there will be times when I will need her to protect me still. And it is of these times I must talk now.

It is a long time since I mentioned the body—too long for a book that is meant to be about that—but the reason for this is a good one: there was much to be said before we could get to here. It is through your body that the true you speaks, but it is also through your body that the other you finds a voice. In the beginning it is difficult to know who is talking, but that does not matter because it is not *why* the body talks that is important here. What is important is the fact that it *does* talk—that and the fact that you *must* listen. It feels right to say it in this way, "you *must* listen", but because of that statement's tone I cannot let it pass without comment. Until now I have been fairly easy going in the way I have talked about things—a take it or leave it approach—but this statement, and in particular the way it is written, signifies a change. The change is one that has occurred in me but that points to, and also requires, a change in you.

There has been a battle going on in this book between the other and the true me. Whenever I have been afraid of moving forward, due to what I'm to say or what you may think, it has been the other me speaking. At the time it worried me that this was the case yet now I realise it had to be this way. Given that the other you is such a big part of who you are, you needed the other me to be present in this book to give you someone to engage with: someone just like you. Without this demonstration of my humanness, I would have been too different and too difficult to relate to.

But you are not the same person as the one who started this book and, having come this far, neither am I. You understand enough about me that my story makes sense and you no longer need me to be the same. I am able to step more fully into the world of the true me and, if you choose, you can follow me into the world of the true you.

50

I've spent a long time thinking about how to listen to the body: whether there are particular thoughts or feelings to look out for and how best to deal with what you hear. As a result of this thinking and my experiences, I'm able to say the following:

Now is the best time to start.
Listen to whatever is there.
Deal with it however you can.

To some of you this may be a let down and, if it is, I'm sorry. I don't have a secret formula or magic trick that's going to make things easy for you. But don't let the simplicity of my words disguise the message that lies beneath:

There is a path available to all of you.
It is an easy one to step upon.

Across the ages one person has led the way and others have followed. It is no different here. In telling my story I'm revealing the existence of a path and encouraging you to take it. I don't want to fall into the trap of prescribing the path itself. To explain what I mean by that consider two of the major religions: Christianity and Buddhism. When Buddha set out, 2,500 years ago, to "teach and communicate his vision"[16], I don't think he had in mind to start a religion. And the same goes for Jesus 500 years later. Both were spiritual people who, having found enlightenment and

God, wanted to share their experiences with others. They did this in the way they lived their lives, how they talked to people and with what they said.

The infrastructures known as Christianity and Buddhism grew up after their deaths and at the hands of their followers. Both were started with the best intentions: to spread the word and give as many people as possible access to the teachings. But in setting down the nature of the way, both ways have become inaccessible to many people. And, more than that, a fundamental truth has been lost: that God is, or enlightenment is, "of its very nature, incommunicable"[17]. Both have to be experienced in order to be known. Being human, the only way God and enlightenment can be experienced is through the body. And also, being human, there's a lot of stuff to get through before we're free enough to experience the divine!

It doesn't matter where you start.
All there needs to be is a beginning.
That is enough.

For me the beginning was not, as you may expect me to say, cancer, but that I listened to my body when it told me what cancer was. It was my way out. It was my escape route. It was my path back to me. And despite cancer's portrayal in the media—always a bad thing but one from which good can sometimes come—I know it has been this way for others too. There are many stories of people for whom cancer has been the turning point in their lives, but this is seen only as a chance by-product of the disease and not as its purpose.

Why do we get cancer? Cancer comes to show us something of ourselves—something we couldn't access in any other way or that would take much longer to access via another route. That cancer has happened to you means there is something for you to learn. There is something important for you to know.

51

We all have the tools needed to listen to the body and act on its advice. It's in getting past the blocks that stop us from doing this that the problems lie. One of the biggest blocks any of us face is fear. Yet most of the time fear is unseen, unacknowledged and, thus, hidden. Cancer is a powerful tool for self-discovery because it brings fear to the surface. Cancer does not create a fear of dying; that fear is already in you, hidden. Cancer brings fear to the surface so that you can deal with it in the open, seeing it for what it is. That you do not want to face your fears and rail against this process is to be expected: you are human and there is nothing wrong in that. It's not how we initially react to cancer that is the problem, but that we get stuck at this point and go no further.

If cancer comes into your life and leaves, without you facing your fear of death and moving past it, a large part of cancer's benefit passes you by. In hiding from death while it is at your door, you not only avoid the fear and upset associated with humanity's view of death, but also miss out on the wonders that lie on the other side of this. But in the beginning the path is difficult—perhaps the most difficult part of the journey—and it's easy to be pushed off course. That's why cancer is, if you allow it to be, such a fantastic companion in those early days. If you acknowledge the issues it raises and deal with them tirelessly and ceaselessly, this in itself will keep you on the path.

In the beginning cancer *is* the path.
It is not the thing from which you must escape.
It is the road to be followed.
And the lamp that lights the way.

Eventually you will reach the point where it is time to part company with cancer. However, in the beginning cancer should be seen, not as the enemy, but as the guide. Just this one change in emphasis is incredibly powerful and can mean the difference between a painful, terrible experience and an extraordinary, life-changing one. But be warned. Those around you may not be so keen on your change of perspective or, to put it another way, your change of heart. Seeing cancer in this way challenges the very foundations of our lives and most people do not want this. As a result some people may try to undermine you—not maliciously or consciously, but this is what they will do. This is not a bad thing for it shows who you can trust. Not everybody will react badly: some will embrace what you have to say and allow themselves to be pulled forward into the world of the true you; while others will simply hold back their views and allow you to be. Both are helpful and nurturing.

I'll share with you the reactions of two of my friends to my way of being with cancer. The first story concerns one of my most spiritual friends, someone who has, without fail, kept pace with me throughout my journey. My friend came to visit one evening a few days after I was diagnosed. She knew I had cancer because we'd spoken on the telephone. When I opened the door she stood there looking tentative and clutching a box of chocolates: 'Celebration' chocolates. As I let her in she explained that, based on what I'd said, a celebration seemed appropriate and that she was going along with it, however strange it felt for her to do so.

Recounting this story brings tears to my eyes: how amazing it is for someone to truly listen to the words of another and do something for that person that feels, not only strange, but that goes against convention and could so easily be misinterpreted. Cancer reveals people's true nature, something that's difficult to discover in normal circumstances: people have had lots of practice at hiding themselves, you see. You have to take someone outside their box to see what they're really made of, and cancer does that for all concerned.

My other friend is German. She lives in Berlin but when I was diagnosed she lived on my street. She is straight-talking, not like English people at all, and you know exactly where you are with her. I remember talking to her between the planned and the actual mastectomy, she said: "I think you've done the wrong thing by refusing the mastectomy. I'm worried you don't know what you're doing, but it's your life and what you do is up to you."

By letting her views be known my friend 'cleared the air' between us and we were able to continue with our friendship despite our difference of opinion. Indeed, I felt closer to my friend *because* of what she'd said. Whether a person speaks her truth or not, it is present in the conversation, or the silences, and can be picked up on. By making feelings known, it's possible for both people to acknowledge them, deal with them and move on. Had my friend not spoken out loud, she'd have been unable to move past her view that I was in the wrong and so, in her eyes, this is where I would have remained.

I want to go back to my friend with the Celebration chocolates. I've remembered something about my feelings at the time and it's important for me to share this with you. It was not only strange for my friend that she brought the chocolates, but strange for me too. Until then the reaction to my euphoria had been as you might expect: people stood back from it and let me be—my strength of feeling and my energy were so strong they could do nothing else. Some were waiting for things to calm down before talking to me, while others didn't know how to behave around me. The reaction of my friend was different. Instead of holding me at arm's length she walked forward and embraced me and, with the chocolates, pushed me forward into the space I'd entered via cancer. Through her actions my friend showed who I was being and this—maybe the enormity of it— brought me down to earth.

Euphoria is all very well but it can only get you so far. It acknowledges, celebrates and raises the spirit but the real work is to be done in the human world, especially with cancer, a disease of the physical. And for that it is necessary to be grounded—and this is what cancer does to most people in the early stages: brings them down to earth with a tremendous bump. No longer can you live in the world of dreams, the world of your imagination, the world of the other you—instead you've to deal with reality.

52

I reacted to cancer as I did partly because I love reality. I can feel it in my body—in the marrow of my bones—and it's from being in touch with reality that I find happiness. I also see the bigger picture first and then go through the emotional trauma and pain, whereas with most people it's the other way round. My way of dealing with things always surprises my friend, the artist. She's amazed at how quickly I move through issues and come out the other side smiling.

Tackling things back-to-front, so to speak, is key to my success. If you know why something has happened and how much you'll grow as a result of it, hurt is easier to deal with. If you have to go through the hurt in order to understand, it's a much more difficult path. Imagine a long journey through rough terrain, full of dark nights and windswept, rain-filled days. If all you see on the horizon is more of the same it's pretty hard going, but if what you see ahead is the Emerald City, that in itself spurs you on and gives the journey purpose and meaning. It's because we don't understand *why* things happen that makes them hard to deal with. Why don't we understand why? Because we look through the eyes of the other you.

The other you doesn't like cancer. Of course it doesn't! Cancer is out to get the other you. At the very least it aims to silence this person and at best it aims to kill them off, leaving the true you in charge of your body. And because you spend a large portion of your time as the other you, cancer is seen as the enemy. But I've said that a few times now, albeit across the book and in a number of ways, so it's time to move on. You need to listen to your body and through that process develop a relationship with the true you.

Only the true you can see things differently.
Only as the true you can you begin to *know*.

Let's go back to what I said about listening to your body: now is the best time to start; listen to whatever is there; deal with it however you can. What are you going to listen to? Why, the cancer of course! Because cancer is the loudest and most urgent of your body's communications, you must start there.

Identifying possible questions

To give the listening focus you need to ask a question relating to your cancer. It may be that a question jumps out at you, that there are a number of possible questions, or that none spring to mind. Each of these is fine.

If one question jumps out at you, you're probably ready for the next step. However, be sure to ask the right type of question, i.e. one that is open. Try not to ask a question that demands a 'yes' or 'no' answer, as it tends to be too limiting. One of the aims of the questioning process is to open you up and this is best achieved with an open question. That said, if you're absolutely convinced that a specific closed question is the right one for you, then ask it.

If you've not identified a question consider these: Why am I afraid to die? Why me? Why do I have cancer? Why cancer and not something else? Choose one using the method below or use them to generate others.

What to consider when selecting a question

If you have a number of possible questions, either from the above list or from your own list, bear in mind the following when selecting the question to be used:

1)   Don't get hung up on choosing the right question. The right question is the one that's right for you in this moment. If you did this exercise on a different day, a different question could be the right one. This is an exercise you can return to at any time.

2)   Choose the question you want to choose and not the one you think you should choose. Don't let someone else choose the question for you. This is your life and you have to take responsibility for it.

3)   Don't be afraid to choose a question that seems silly or irrelevant. These often give the most powerful results. If you want to ask, "Why do I always think of my cancer as purple?" then ask it. Similarly with, "Why is it that every time I think about my cancer I'm reminded of that strange bird I saw on holiday?" Don't let anything stop you asking the question you want to ask.

4)   Finally, and most importantly, choose your question with your body and not with your mind. Your mind is useful in drawing up a list of questions but should not be used to select a question from that list. Your mind is too influenced by the world of the other you to select on the basis of truth.

While your body is guided only by your inner wisdom, your mind bases its decision-making on the factors it's been told to take account of. It's a computer that, since birth, has been programmed by you, your parents, your peers and society. If you ask your mind, "which question?" it will come up with an answer based on the information available to it.

It will choose on the basis of what the other you knows and what the other you considers to be important.

When you ask your body, "which question?" it chooses only with guidance from the true you. In this way your body draws you closer to your truth. But that aside, as it's your body that's given you cancer it's to your body you should be looking for answers.

Selecting and answering questions

The process for selecting a question with your body is the same as for answering the question itself:

1)   **Frame the process of enquiry with a question.** When selecting a question, the question is "which question?" By specifying your question you are stating the objective of the exercise.

2)   **Put your question to one side.** Having asked your question, immediately forget about it. You need to do this to create a space for your question to be answered with your body and not with your mind. When I do this I have a mental picture in which I lift the question and move it to one side. Some of you may find it helpful to physically imitate this movement, i.e. to imagine yourself picking up the question with your hands and moving it out of your range of vision.

3)   **Step inside your body.** This requires that you place your consciousness inside your body. My consciousness always starts from a place outside of my body and a little in front of it. I move my consciousness into my body using my eyes; they map the arc it makes as I step inside. Do whatever works for you to bring awareness into your body.

4)   **Describe and explore what's there.** This is both the most difficult and the easiest part of the process. It's easy because you simply follow the lead of your body, using

your senses to explore what you find, i.e. you look, listen, touch, taste and smell. It's difficult because you must let thoughts arise in support of the process but at the same time allow them to pass through—and in this way it's akin to meditation.

There will be times in the process where questions arise or where thoughts start to form in answer to your initial question. The key is to not get caught up in these. If this does happen, eventually you will become aware that you are thinking and have stepped outside your body and into your head. In such cases, simply step back inside your body, i.e. go back to step 3, and start again from there.

Don't worry if your thoughts continually distract you or your attention is diverted by something else. I've taken 'phone calls in the middle of this process and have even stopped for lunch. It's easy to restart the process: simply go back to where you left off.

To help with re-starting and with the process in general, it's best to write down what you find. The examples I give later in the chapter will help you with this but basically it's easy: you write what you see, or feel, or hear, or taste, or smell, and what you are doing.

5)   **Continue until you have an answer.** There will come a point where an answer becomes clear. I say "an answer", because sometimes the enquiry reveals a larger truth that makes the original question, and thus its answer, irrelevant. That's fine. In fact, it's great. The purpose of the process is not to find an answer to a specific question, but to move forward into the unknown and closer to your truth. If you can fast-track in the way I've described, all well and good.

In terms of knowing the answer, it's the bodily *knowing* you're waiting for; the one I've talked about in various parts of the book. It exists in your body and not in your head, and often resides in the place between your belly button and your heart.

To help you understand the process I'll share my experience of it. Because I'd not developed this tool when I had cancer—getting closer to my truth was much more hit and miss—I don't have anything I can share with you from that time. And as I don't have any cancer-related questions that remain unanswered, I can't use that route either. Therefore, to demonstrate how the process works I'll start with, "which question?" This makes perfect sense, as it will be here that some of you begin.

(Before I start, I'll head for the loo and make a cup of tea—although stopping and starting is fine, it's best to think ahead a little!)

Using your body to identify a question (example)

I frame the process of enquiry with "which question?" (I feel the need to state that I do not know what the question, and therefore the answer, might be.)

I step inside my body. I stand inside my torso, in my stomach; in the place between my belly button and my heart, where the knowing comes from. I feel slightly nervous. Is this a fear that the process will not work? I allow that question to pass through and come back to my stomach.

I feel something in the underside of my chin, in the soft bit just along from the top of my neck. It is a slight pressure. In my head it feels as if awareness is beginning to grow. It is as if part of my consciousness has moved up to my head and that from here the answer will come. I have a feeling of anticipation.

I am distracted by something. A picture wants to form in my mind. I was remembering that, previously during this exercise, I have seen shapes and the distraction came from there.

The anticipation has moved to my torso and sits on top of my diaphragm. I am chasing something all over my body! I feel stuck. The thought, "I'm chasing the answer", came to mind and as it departed left me feeling solid. This feeling has replaced the feeling of anticipation on the top of my diaphragm.

Doubts start to creep in: "Is this rubbish? Is this going to work?" But I see these as doubts and they go away. The knowing is here. It sits in that soft place under my chin. It feels as if it is smiling at me in a knowing way—as knowing would, I suppose! It has something to do with "which question?"

I become aware of a slight ache at the bottom of my cheeks, the kind that would exist as a remnant of a clenched jaw. The base of my neck at the top of my back aches and suddenly I feel close to tears. There is a pain in my chest where my left breast once was and I think, "this must be significant". But the pain disappears and is replaced with a headache, joining the ache in my neck. The ache in my cheeks has dropped down my jaw, and is in the soft place under my chin. This makes me think of vulnerability.

Why am I so vulnerable?
The question emerges.

That's how the process works. It's that simple. The key is to stick with it, report what's there and keep going until an answer emerges. You may not be able to write down all your thoughts, they may be too fleeting, but you will need to report them if they get stuck in your mind and stop you moving on. I wrote: "I am distracted by something...I was remembering that previously during this exercise I have seen shapes and the distraction came from there." Only when the memory began to distract me did I need to acknowledge it consciously in order to move on. This is where writing helps. Recording thoughts acknowledges them in a physical way and makes them easier to let go of. Writing also makes you give clear descriptions of what you find. It is, therefore, an integral part of the process.

Having found my question it's time to answer it. However it's late in the day, I feel tired and I'm going to leave it for tomorrow. This also gives me the opportunity to say the following: I have no desire to think about the question, nor will I try to answer it overnight. I do not need to set my brain to work on this. My body will give me the answer in the morning. And more than that, any answers my brain came up with would just get in the way tomorrow. They would push for my attention during the process and make it more difficult. So I'll forget about the question until tomorrow. Talk to you then.

I'm back, not one but three days later: a pipe burst at my son's school and it was closed for two days. While initially frustrating, the time out has been good for both of us. My son needed time with his mum and I've had the opportunity to see the effect of having a 'true you' question unanswered for so long. I *need* to have the question answered. The energy that has built up in my body needs to be given voice and dissipated.

The first night, I went to bed with little thought of vulnerability—indeed I'm still giving it little thought—it's not my mind that the issue is preoccupying but my body.

It's pressing for my attention and has been since yesterday. Today the pressure to answer the question has become almost unbearable. The pressure is driven from the area below my belly button, from the place in Tai Chi called the Tan Tien, or the energy centre of the body. It feels as if there is an active volcano inside me with pressure building at my neck. I can delay no more. I must answer the question. As before, I do not know—indeed I have no idea—what the answer will be.

Answering a question with the body (example)

Why am I so vulnerable? As soon as I ask the question I feel a prick of tears and a sense of relief. There is no need to step inside my body as my consciousness is already inside. It wants the question to be answered.

I become aware of a sensation in the area below my belly button. It no longer feels as if this area is driving the volcano; indeed the volcano has disappeared. What I feel instead is energy, concentrated into an area the size of a small orange. (I make a shape with my hands to judge the size that is right.)

Why am I so vulnerable? The question pops into my head to remind me what the process is for.

The orange-sized energy is swirling in the area below my belly button; not quickly, but at the speed one would use if stirring a sauce while cooking. This analogy relaxes me slightly and I feel somewhat happier. It is as if I have dropped down a level and am getting closer to the truth. I am aware of two doors that want to shut. I cannot see a picture of these in my mind but they are there—behind me and a little to the right of the back of my head. They are the part of me that does not want to see but, in this instance, this part is not strong.

I try to return to my body, but still I feel the draw of that area behind my head. There is something for me to see here, something that is close to me but due to its location remains hidden from view. I wonder if I can move it into my vision, and with that I feel the beginnings of a lump in my throat and I step closer to tears. Is this because I am now ready to see? The question stops the process and I feel harder, colder and less vulnerable. Less vulnerable. This is important. There is something about the process of—no, the experience of—vulnerability that, that...I do not have the words. It is something to do with needing to be this way to see life for what it is. Tears are one step closer still.

My head butts in. "I know this!" At some level I know this and my intellect is trying to help me. But that is not the way. That can never be the way for me. I do what I must do and return to my body, back to that place below MY BELLY BUTTON. For some reason MY CONSCIOUS NESS wants me to be there. This is how the words were typed, in my hurry I somehow hit the caps lock button. My subconscious really is trying to tell me something! The area below the belly button is important, as is conscious [space] ness. Is there something in that space? It feels important but I can't see how or why.

I return to the place below my belly button and am glad to be returning there. Glad in a 'what a relief' way and not a joyful one. Maybe I should sit here for a while. I put my hand below my belly button to see if it helps. It doesn't. The feeling of my hand on the outside of my body distracts from the need to be inside. We need to be inside our bodies, but this makes us vulnerable. We need to be vulnerable. Why am I vulnerable? "Because I need to be."

But this is not enough. I cannot stop here. This is not the end. Why do I need to be vulnerable? This becomes the question. "Because!" shouts a voice in my head—but it is not the voice of my head, it is the voice of my body inside my head and this is not the same. The voice of the body inside the head is more inside the head, somehow, than the voice of the mind. I think of schizophrenics but have to shut that down. The answer does not lay there.

Why do I need to be vulnerable? I step inside my body, again to that place below my belly button. It feels different though. It feels spongy. It is as if I could knead it like dough with my feet or my hands. It does not look like dough nor is it the same consistency; it has no physicality and yet, somehow, it feels like dough. There are no edges to it. It has no beginning and no end. It simply exists. "Like our souls", my head interjects. I am becoming impatient with how long this is taking, but tell myself there is a reason why. I am drawn back to the dough and ask again: "Why do I need to be vulnerable?" That voice comes again, "Because!" But it is fainter than last time. I must stop asking the question. It is taking me away from the truth.

Inside my body, that's where I want to be.
My body wants to type that, with no recourse to me.
Inside my body, is the place for all to see...

My head butted in to write the last line, and so interrupted the poetry. I return to my body. My consciousness has moved slightly higher in my body. Is my consciousness being raised? It sits on top of my diaphragm. I remember that from this place previously the answer came. I have a—that same?—feeling of anticipation. My mind is empty and I am grateful for that. The top of my diaphragm is flat;

a sheet of something sits on it, smooth to the touch. I feel the need for my head to butt in: "Go away head!" I run my hand across the surface of the sheet. This will keep me where I need to be. That makes me angry. There is so much of that 'keeping us where we need to be'.

The sheet has the answer. I stroke the surface of it. It is grey like metal but feels like plastic—no, more like a mineral. I am reminded of something my counsellor said yesterday: "When we die our souls are released and our mineral body dies." (I get a glimpse of where I am going with this and a tingle runs though my body, top to bottom.) "But in some way our physical body does not die because what we learn from it stays with our souls for all eternity." So come on Lesley! (I start to get tough with myself.) We need to be vulnerable because? This is the only way we can learn. But this is a head-based answer and again not enough.

Back to the mineral sheet. It is thin, almost wafer thin, but it is strong. I am reminded of our bodies and how thin, i.e. how open to injury, they are and yet they are strong. There is something in being human that makes us strong. It is the very vulnerability of our bodies that makes us strong. I am a few steps closer to tears. I try to go back to the sheet but things have moved on and this no longer helps. It is something about the very nature of flesh, of skin, of tissue—of something that can be cut with a knife. Our souls are eternal, inviolable and yet they reside in something so vulnerable. Why is that?

I return to my body. My consciousness is in my throat. I feel a pressure there. It is slight. It is concentrated. It is my body preparing to speak. I open my mouth in the hope that this will help. It does not. I return to my throat. It is about giving voice. The body gives voice to the soul. Vulnerability gives the body?...Vulnerability gives the soul?...

Back to my body. Now my consciousness is in my chest, in my heart chakra. It feels as if it is concentrating itself, ready to make a leap. I need to focus on it as it shrinks. I need to tie myself into the concentrating process. If I can do this, then I will know. It loses nothing of itself when it shrinks. It is shrinking physically but in no other way. (I must shut up my head, which is reaching like an octopus with many tentacles, searching for the answer.) It is the size of a pinprick, my consciousness—no, the size of a pea. It is becoming a pinprick and I anticipated that.

I realise I am typing too fast. Not looking at what I'm writing. Wanting to rush the process. I slow myself. I start to pay attention to the writing and to the spelling. This is important as it gives the brain something to do. It keeps it occupied while the real work is done elsewhere.

I can see my consciousness no more. I cannot look with my eyes and need to look into my body with another sense: my *knowing* or my intuition. Using this, my consciousness has no shape—I am not using my eyes, how could it have shape?—but my consciousness is there. I look down, as if I am looking with my throat: a direct connection between body and truth. I sit for a while and allow myself to be. Being forceful is the problem. It has to stop.

My consciousness sits between my belly button and my heart, in the place where the knowing comes from. It is happy there. It is a good place for it to be. It has chosen this place—tears well up—above all others. I feel the joy of my consciousness, of my soul. It is the happiness I explained before, happiness that fills you from the inside out. It comes not from the body but from the soul. Through the body we get to experience the soul. We get to feel the soul and know its beauty and its wonders. I am overtaken by my desire to communicate this and it shuts down the words.

I glimpse something. A pause for sobbing, for drying my eyes. I put my head in my hands and sob some more. The soul is happy here because here it can be known. *Knowing* is knowing the soul. In your body your soul can know itself. It can see itself through your eyes, through the eyes of a vulnerable human being.

Is the question of vulnerability answered? I do not know. But if I take a break to edit the text and get a cup of tea, then I will know. From previous experience of the process I know what this time is for. There needs to be time for the things I have discovered to diffuse—to grow—out of my soul and into my body and take their place there. They need to become part of me—of my physicality—before I can move on.

It's some time later and I'm back. I've finished editing (mainly correcting spelling and grammar), I've had my lunch and I'm on my second cup of tea. I've reached the point where I am ready to speak. I do not need to return to the exercise. The words I need are present in my body (although I do not yet know what they are) and I do not need to look for them. The exercise has brought me to the place where I can access my truth.

Your soul—the true you—is all things. By its very nature it is truth; it is love; it is joy. It has chosen to be human to experience these qualities and give them life and expression. Your body shrouds the soul and breaks the soul's contact with itself, so giving the soul your body's eyes. The soul experiences though the body, and the body gives depth and meaning to the soul qualities. Thus love is experienced in human form: as the love of a mother for her child; as the love of a man for his wife; as the love of music; as the love of poetry; and as the love of landscape. And perhaps more importantly, love is experienced as the absence of love. To the light, life gives the experience of shade.

53

Using the process described in the last chapter you will gain access to your truth: in this case the truth of your cancer. What you uncover will probably not be what you expect, and it may not be easy to deal with. But because it is truth it has the power to transform your life, and it will do just that—if you allow it to. You do not have to take the path I am offering and that will be revealed to you through your body—the choice remains yours. If you decide to take the path, you need to know that the longer you follow it the harder it will be to turn away; eventually you will reach a point where there is no turning back; where it is the path or nothing.

The day I was diagnosed with cancer I chose my path. This was made easy for me because I first found the path when my husband left, but then I lost it; I had experienced the emptiness of life without it. Having, again, found the path with cancer, I refused to let it go. Even the threat of death was not enough to make me turn. For me, therefore, choosing my path and the point of no return coincided. For most people this is not the case, but for me it had to be this way. Without this coincidence, I could not have written this book. It is because these two events came together that my path has been, from the beginning, clear. And because of this, I have something to say.

There is power in both the choosing of the path and in the point of no return, and when these events coincide their power is multiplied. The euphoria I felt as I left the hospital on the day of diagnosis was my body's reaction to this power.

What is this power?
It is the experience of God.

When you first choose the path, and when you choose the path over all other paths, you are choosing the path to God and so allowing God to enter your life. This does not mean, when you consider the path, it has to be about God. God is my word to describe what I feel; it does not have to be yours. Indeed, you can follow the path and get all you need from it, simply by paying attention to the feelings generated in your body. Unless, via the questioning of your body, you have identified a specific action—and for most people this will not be the case—your next step is to sit with what has been uncovered and wait for the path to be further revealed. This requires both patience and trust—qualities most people need to develop, me included.

The choice you face is the path of the true you versus the path of the other you. Or to put it another way, choosing to be led by your truth instead of by what the outside world holds true. If you choose your true path above that of the other you, you may experience conflict in the external world. If you choose the path of the other you over your true path, you will experience internal conflict. It is interesting how many of us choose to suffer internally, rather than to face conflict with others.

Internal conflict takes many forms—from feelings of unhappiness, through emotional illnesses such as depression, right up to severe physical illness such as cancer—but, confusingly, this conflict is not restricted to the internal world. Because we do not live in isolation, internal conflict leaks into the external world through our interactions with others. Indeed, it is via this mechanism that the world of the other you is created. The external world is simply a manifestation of our individual internal struggles. It stands to reason, therefore, that as we change ourselves so we change the world. However hard that may be for you to believe—looking at it through the eyes of the other you—I know this to be true. If you want to change the world, look inside. The answers and the means lay there.

How conflict manifested itself for me during cancer was in my dealings with the medical profession and some of my family, particularly my mum and dad. (Before cancer almost all my conflict had been internal: my workaholism, my depression and a tendency to hide myself away.) Owing to science, belief and duty, doctors have a clear and often narrow view of what is best for a cancer patient. The degree to which their suggested path and your actual path overlap should depend entirely on you. My mind has returned to the day of the diagnosis, to the moment when the cancer was revealed. I'm sitting in the doctor's office, him behind the desk, me in front, and the breast-care nurse to one side. The results of my tests lay on the desk and the doctor speaks. "I'm sorry to tell you, you have breast cancer. You'll need to have an operation."

"Only if I want one."

My reaction surprised him and after a pause, he said: "Of course, only if you want one."

My five words, and in particular the energy with which they were delivered, defined the nature of the interaction between us. Normally the doctor would have been in control of the discussion, but with those five words I turned things on their head and control came back to me. And that's how it should be.

This is your body.
This is your cancer.

This is your life.

While others can provide counsel, the decisions must be made by you. But let's get back to my reaction. It surprised me, it was spontaneous, and it was out before I'd registered it.

It's the energy of the words that's important: it's not so much what was said, as how it was said that made the difference. I'm reminded of the story in Chapter 8, where I changed a request to meet the needs of another instead of my own. Then, it was the other person's tone of voice that caused the change, but the changes that took place in the doctor's office were not initiated by that — there was no anger or upset in my voice. The power came not from any manipulation on my part, but from the energy with which the words emerged. The words came from the true me and it is this that gave them power.

In the world of the other you very little is true — by that I do not mean that things are false, although they sometimes are, but that the world is not an expression of the truth that lies within us. Instead, the world is made up of material facts, i.e. facts relating to the physical world, and expressions of the other you. Paradise, as I see it, would be a world made up of material facts and expressions of the true you.

Both the true you and the other you have the power to change the world. When you are being the true you, you change the world simply as a result of being that person: you don't have to do anything, save for being yourself. As you speak and act out your truth, so it gives others access to their truth and it is via this mechanism — and this mechanism alone — that the world is changed.

When you are being the other you it's more complex.

There are many more ways in which you can change the world, all of which are a form of manipulation. At one extreme is killing another to get what you want; at the other is withholding your truth in order to fit in. In between are the countless other ways in which we fail to be true: the grumpiness, the jealousy, the little white lies; bullying, alcohol abuse and infidelity; theft, physical abuse and rape. All of these are manifestations of the internal struggle that comes from being the other you.

54

Cancer is not punishment for the other you, it is a consequence of *being* this person. To remain healthy our bodies need to be imbued with life force: the energy that comes from connection with and manifestation of our divinity (the true you). If you are out of touch with this life force for too long, you become ill. If you do not reconnect with it, you die. This life force is what we know as, and what we recognise as, life.

I am reminded of a walk by the river when my son was a toddler. It was springtime and life was in the process of renewal. The river runs through the city and the concrete banks are high, as much as 20 feet in parts. The river meanders but the landscape is angular. The banks are sheer and form a series of straight lines that approximate the curve of the river.

We always stopped at the same place, where the line of the bank is broken by a right-angled turn into the bank, then another to correct its path. In the slack waters created by the turn is a set of wide, shallow-treaded steps built into the concrete. These lead down through the surface of the water to the riverbed. To the right of the steps as you sit on them is a slope giving access to the water for small craft. To the left, the bank is wider where it turns and is often taken by anglers. That day my son and I were alone. There are houses close by—separated from the river by a footpath, a narrow road and small, town gardens. The area is popular with people walking into the city, but at that time of day— late morning, but before the lunchtime rush—it was empty, save for us.

On the wide bank close to the steps lay a duckling, only a few days old. Its feathers were soft-yellow and fine enough that its body shape could be made out beneath them. The duckling lay outstretched, beak and feet as far apart as they could be. It was dead, laid out as if by a human hand. As soon as I saw the duckling I knew it was dead. Not because there were signs of death—there was no broken skin, no blood, no loss of feathers—or because there was an absence of life signs—the duckling did not move, but that was not it. I knew the duckling was dead because what I know to be life—what I recognise as life—was not present. In the absence of life I saw, for the first time, what life is.

55

Being the true you changes the world because it calls into being those around you. When the true you shines, it does so for all to see. In the presence of life as it is meant to be lived—in the presence of truth and God—the other you within yourself and others is revealed. Revelation is what interests and excites me about the human condition. It's also this—or rather the outcome of this—that keeps me on my path and stops me turning back.

I need to talk about this 'no turning back'. Unless I elaborate on it, this aspect of the path may stop some of you from taking it. It would be easy to look at no turning back in a physical sense and to view it as an outcome of burning my bridges, i.e. giving up my job and selling my house, but it is not about that. It's not that there is no route back—I was offered work just a month ago—but that I do not want to take it. And more than that, I have changed so much I am no longer able to take it. The inability to turn back is not a negative thing. It comes, not from a narrowing of choice, but from increasing awareness and personal growth. I am unable to turn back because I know what would be required and I am not prepared to do it. It would demand shutting down my truth, denying my uniqueness and hiding myself away. To go back would require that I stop being me and I stop being true. I cannot do that.

You, thanks to cancer, are at a point of revelation. At such a point there are but two paths you can follow: one is the path of truth, the other the path of illusion. The path of truth requires that you accept your situation, seeing it for what it is, and that you make changes in your life based on what you see. This is a difficult path and presents many challenges. The path of illusion requires that you change nothing, but this in itself is an illusion, because in the light of revelation you need to work harder simply to maintain the status quo. Although it appears to be the easier option, the path of illusion is, in the long run, the more difficult one.

Revelation *is* light and it highlights aspects of your life that need to change. To follow the path of truth requires only that you look at and allow yourself to be with what is revealed, acting on it when you are ready and able. If you choose—consciously, but more often unconsciously—not to follow the path of truth, the path of illusion is the only one open to you. All paths that are not the path of truth are the path of illusion. To follow the path of illusion in the light of revelation requires action. You must either extinguish the light—as happened when I let the know-it-alls get to me—or you must hide it. There are many ways to hide the light, all of which give rise to the other you.

When I postponed my mastectomy I was, if you remember, waiting—although I didn't know it—for the point where I could no longer go back to my old life. This was reached when I talked to my mum and dad about feeling unloved as a child, and this is what I said about it in Chapter 47: "That my parents didn't love me was not true, but in my world—the world of the other me—I believed this and therefore it was true to me. I don't know why the speaking of this 'imagined truth' made a difference, but this is surely what it did." I now understand why this was so important. That my parents did not love me was the oldest and biggest part of the other me. Once I spoke of it and its existence was revealed, it could be seen by us and became real. Until that point I had concealed this aspect of the other me from them, hiding within her in order to feel right with the world. As soon as this part of the other me was seen and became real, she was no longer part of my world of illusion. Thus, this world began to crumble.

Since that time my path has revealed many aspects of the other me—some I have let go of, others I still hold. Because many of my other me personas have dropped away, fewer paths of illusion are available to me. This, combined with my developing consciousness—every time a part of the other you is dropped, consciousness increases—helps keep me on the path of truth. I am hoping that for you, this book will be the light. That sufficient of your other you personas will be revealed, enabling you to take the path of truth: it is not enough that you want to take it, you must be ready to take it also. It is so easy for the energy of revelation to be lost—for it to be buried underneath, or consumed by, the other you—and the more other you personas you have, the more likely it is that the energy will be dissipated. And without this energy, change is impossible.

56

I want to talk about something we can all relate to: food and drink. When we overeat or eat foods that are bad for us, or when we drink to achieve a specific outcome, we are adopting an other you persona to hide from the truth. There are many reasons why we do this, most of which are hidden from view.

Even after a year, almost to the day, on my 'can't eat anything that normal people eat' diet, I'm still struggling with it. The problem isn't the diet itself, but that I use food to stop myself seeing things as they are. This isn't a conscious thing—how could it be given what I'm committed to? But it is a well-established pattern. However, yesterday I saw how I use food as a hiding place, and I hope this will help me to change. Instead of looking at the habit itself—feeling hungry all the time and eating too much—I looked at what was happening in terms of my body's energy, using the exercise in Chapter 52. I asked the question: "What is this feeling of restlessness?" Although I didn't get an answer— it's not always about that—I did get rid of the feeling and had the following insights. Another case of life, or rather my body, giving me what I need for this book.

I'll begin by going back a few months: very rarely do insights come out of the blue. That day I'd sent a letter to a literary agent and the experience left me feeling uneasy. I wasn't worried, as such, about contacting the agent, nor was I excited. However, it was a 'big thing' and this registered in my body as a surplus of energy. The energy was uncomfortable to be with and, as there seemed to be nowhere for this feeling to go, I ate it away with chocolate. This was, unusually, a deliberate act. I said to one of the mums from school, "I'm going to buy some chocolate because it's the only way I'm going to get my energy down."

I lay on the sofa, eating the chocolate, savouring every mouthful. While the chocolate did as I'd hoped—it took my energy down to a level where I could cope with it and, therefore, took away the uneasy feeling—it also had an unexpected side effect. As soon as I finished the chocolate a headache and a fog appeared in my head, making it difficult for me to think straight or to see clearly, not in a physical sense (my eyesight was unaffected) but mentally, i.e. I lost my mental clarity. Why did this happen? It always happens, it's just that most of the time we don't notice. But my system was clean—that's the aim of my diet, after all— and because of that I was aware of the chocolate's effect.

Everything we eat or drink impacts on us, but most of the time we do not see what that impact is. The main exception is alcohol: we know the effect it has on our bodies, both good and bad. We know that when we start to drink we feel relaxed and sociable, but that if we drink too much we lose the ability to think straight and stand upright—amongst other things! Most people learn to use alcohol so that it gives what is required without the nasty side effects, i.e. we learn to ration ourselves, not many get to the point where they are weaned from it as I was.

It's interesting to see the letting go of the other you as weaning. In the beginning the other you is necessary, but there comes a time when you have to move on from it if you are to become all that you can be; like a child moving from milk to pureed solids to other easy-to-digest foods so, as you grow, you swap one aspect of the other you for another. In our late teens and early twenties alcohol is useful in social situations. It gives us confidence and enables us to interact with new people, let go of our worries and enjoy ourselves. Yet alcohol is but a hiding place, concealing from view the parts of ourselves that get in the way of a good night out. If you can't enjoy yourself without alcohol, you can't enjoy yourself as you are. But, as I said above, alcohol is different from many other you personas, in that when we drink most of us know what we're doing and why. The personas I'm interested in are the ones that affect us more subtly, at the energy level. These we pull over our heads like invisible jumpers, unseen by both the wearer and others.

Overeating, eating the wrong things and under-eating all stem from the need to balance energy within the body—rather than addressing the root cause of the imbalance we mask it or mend it with food. While the body is busy digesting, adjusting blood sugar levels and detoxifying, it has little energy remaining to communicate our truth to us. Overloading or starving the body is a good way to shut it up! Your body complains about the food or lack of it, but while it's doing that it isn't nagging you about other things—not so that you can hear it anyhow. The other you uses food to dissipate energy that is needed elsewhere, i.e. for emotional and spiritual growth. Eating the wrong things, at the wrong times and in the wrong amounts stops the natural process of development and enlightenment. We are meant to thrive and grow. Misuse of food is just one of the ways in which the other you is expert at stopping this process.

Today for lunch I had a large green salad: two types of lettuce plus rocket and watercress, with cucumber, mango, avocado and smoked tofu. I finished my meal with a large slice of banana tofu cheesecake (wheat, dairy and sugar-free). My body does not need food. I am not empty or lacking in nutrition. But still I feel hungry some of the time. I dip into hunger as I lose touch with my current state of being and out of it as I reconnect. When I am present, i.e. in my body, I feel the energy in my body and the associated emotion. I am also in touch with my full stomach and am not hungry. The hunger returns as my awareness of myself disappears.

I am at a pivot point—imagine a seesaw moving slowly on its pivot—shifting in and out of two states of being. Feeling the existence of the pivot is important. Being wholly in one state of being or the other brings only an experience of that one state. Switching between two states gives an experience of both and with this comes awareness and understanding. At this pivotal point I can see what shifts me between unreal hunger and contentment, and this knowledge gives me the ability to switch out of unreal hunger when that feeling comes. Without this knowledge my options are narrowed to eating more, or to denial—the pattern so many of us fall into when it comes to food. We eat too much: we diet (denial). We eat too much: we diet (denial). We switch between two responses to our energy imbalances, neither of which address or even acknowledge the root cause.

57

The fight against cancer is a fight against you. A battle is taking place in your body between your immune system and the cancerous cells. This mimics the battle between the true you and the other you. If the cancer is to be defeated, so must the other you. The other you gains strength in hiding. Unaware of it, you give it the energy it needs to survive and grow. If you bring the other you out into the open and see it for what it is—part of you but not your truth—you can let it go. The key to this is your body. It will communicate the existence of the other and the true you at every available opportunity and in every way it can. All you need do is pay attention and listen to what it has to say.

The exercise in Chapter 52 provides a means of eliciting information from the body, but the information of interest here is that which the body volunteers. You're looking for those occasions when the other you shows itself, i.e. for times when your internal conflicts leak out into the world. Your body will draw attention to these by the way it makes you feel. Feeling hungry when you've eaten enough is one such communication. If, like me, you eat too much and then feel bad about it, this is also a communication from the body. Emotions reveal an aspect of the other you, either in yourself or others. The difficulty lies in catching an emotion as it arises and seeing it for what it is: communication. This is not easy as we tend to get drawn into the emotion and allow it to dominate. This is a hard habit to break but as with everything, you simply need a place to start.

My mind is taken back to a conversation with my acupuncturist. It took place two years ago. I was complaining about difficulties in getting to sleep—a recurrent theme. She suggested that before going to bed I have a relaxing bath and pamper myself. When she said this I could see I had a problem, revealed to me by my reaction to her suggestion: I was repulsed by it, so much so that I almost shuddered and grimaced. Because the feeling was so strong and completely out-of-line with a normal response to her suggestion, I knew I had to look at it; it had to be masking something I did not want to see. It didn't take long to identify the issue. A relationship of four months had ended abruptly a few weeks before and, rather than dealing with it, I was ignoring it; keeping myself busy and not allowing time for emotions to surface. My feeling of repulsion was part of the other me, formed to hide the truth: that I was upset, I was hurt and there was healing to do.

When watching for the other you, you're waiting for occasions when it gets so far out-of-line with your truth that it gives itself away. My reaction to the suggestion of a bath was one such instance and my behaviour at the hairdressers (Chapter 10) was another. In both cases the other me revealed itself with emotion: repulsion and fear, respectively. In the case of my hair, this was also accompanied by action: failing to take out of my bag pictures of haircuts I liked and, as a result, ending up with yet another bad haircut. Just as the true you is expressed through your personality, so it is with the other you. The other me is almost always a bit odd—and the same could be said of the true me! Your other you will have its own unique characteristics.

A couple of weeks ago a friend called to talk about work; she'd behaved in a way she was unhappy with and was worried about it. "I'm going off the rails!" she cried.

"No," I replied. "You're like a boxcar that's taken a bend too quickly; you're leaning too far to one side. Two of your wheels are off the tracks but you're still moving in the right direction. It's a warning sign, that's all. There are things you need to look at. Give them the attention they need and all will be well; ignore them and the situation will get worse. There's no harm done, but you do need to sort this out."

As we talked further, the issues became clear. My friend was avoiding taking responsibility for an aspect of her life and because the issues were big and difficult to face, she was hiding from them. To balance this she had, unconsciously, started to take responsibility for someone else's life—and this created the issue at work. The nature of my friend's other-you behaviour gave a clue to her real issue and this is often the case, e.g. my fear of a haircut masked a deeper fear relating to self image.

When faced with other-you behaviour (in yourself or others), the key to uncovering truth is to look at the behaviour dispassionately and not get hung up on it. The aim is to see what has occurred, not from the perspective of the other you, but from the perspective of truth. If you can do this the real issues become clear. This is not to say that other-you behaviour should be ignored, only that you shouldn't beat yourself up for it. Indeed beating yourself up over your actions is simply another aspect of the other you. In the past, if I did something 'wrong' it would take me weeks, maybe months, to get over it—if I got over it at all. I would continually replay events in my head, making myself feel bad and small. We're not talking big things here—remember my other you does not have a very dark side—but minor indiscretions, such as a work-related error or failing to speak my truth. Then one day I had a moment of realisation when, in the middle of beating myself up, I saw that this was simply my way of staying stuck.

Beating myself enabled me to do the same things over and over again, with the only cost being the, albeit painful, reliving of the deeds. The benefit, however, was that I didn't have to move on because I didn't take responsibility for what I'd done. If I never forgave myself I didn't have to own what I'd done or, more importantly, take care to make sure it didn't happen again. There is always a benefit to other you behaviour, however damaging it is to ourselves or to others, and that is why we choose to be the other you. Note: not getting hung up on other you behaviour and not beating yourself up for it does not mean you can ignore the consequences of being the other you. If you commit adultery you could damage a relationship; if you break the law you could go to jail. There are consequences to everything we do and facing up to these is a key part of moving on from the other you.

Getting well will require that you accept and own all that you are, before choosing which bits to keep and which to discard. Facing the truth of who you are—both the other and the true you—is integral to your path back to you and, therefore, integral to good health. In the West we tend to think of being well as not being ill, but being well can be so much more than this. I'm still not well in the way I want to be; although I no longer have cancer and people often say, "you look really well", this is not enough. It's not the fear of being unwell that's driving me forward, but the idea of how I'll feel when I reach my goal. If life feels this good now, how much better it will be when I'm at my best. What are you aiming for with cancer? To return to the health you enjoyed before you fell ill? Or could there be — should there be — more for you?

Being well is a question of balance; not the work-life balance that preoccupies so many of us, but the balance of energy in the body. To be well our physical, emotional, intellectual and spiritual selves need to be in balance, both within themselves and with each other. For a body to be well, it needs more than just a healthy, balanced diet. The physical body is impacted not only by the energy presented to it in food, but also by that arising from our emotions, thoughts and spirit. If emotions are suppressed or repressed, if negative thoughts are allowed to dominate and/or the spirit is denied, the resultant energy will force the body away from health. If such conditions are allowed to continue over a prolonged period of time, the body will become ill. The way back to health is to bring balance back to the body, paying attention to all aspects of ourselves.

The traditional approach to health and wellbeing focuses on one aspect of the self to the exclusion of others. Those wanting physical health improve their diet and exercise more. Those with emotional issues attempt to move past these via counselling, psychotherapy and associated practices. And those looking for spiritual health and growth seek guidance from religion and other sources. But working on one aspect of the self is not enough, for such an approach ignores the interconnectedness between the various parts of the self and their dependence on each other. Looking at the self from the perspective of the other versus the true you offers a different approach. Instead of focusing on one aspect of the self, the path back to health is mapped out by the true you, through the landscape of the other you, using the body as the guide. The path to health is, thus, the path to truth.

The landscape of the other you includes aspects of your physical, emotional and intellectual self. It is a complex and multifaceted landscape and therefore easy to lose yourself in. The route back to health requires that you traverse the landscape in its entirety, become familiar with it and, as a result of your awareness of it, transform it into the landscape of the true you. When the true you begins to take over the landscape, you will begin to be well. The more the true you comes to dominate the landscape, the closer to perfect health and the happier you will be.

Most spiritual paths have been set by religious orders that specify, in quite some detail, the rules of the path. This path is different, in that there are no rules other than the general ones: listen to your body and let the true you lead; watch out for the other you, come to understand it and learn to let it go. No actions are out-of-bounds and there are no moral guidelines. Thus, to all intents and purposes, anything goes. It has to be this way because of the other you. The battle against cancer is fought against the other you, and that person needs to be seen and understood if they are to be beaten.

The landscape of the other you is as it is. It has its dark forests. It has its high mountains. It has its barren plains. And you will need to spend time in all of these places if you are to become well. Pretending they do not exist is not a long-term option, for denial of the truth is just another habitat of the other you. I'm not suggesting that you get lost in the other you or that you allow yourself to be seduced by it, only that you see it for what it is and deal with it accordingly. I cannot tell you the path to take through the landscape of the other you, only how to navigate: with your body. It points the way like a compass taking its direction from—and only from—the true you.

It doesn't matter where you start
Whether you take a wrong turn
Or how many times you stray from the path
There will always be a path back to you.

58

Because the true you guides you through the landscape of the other you, part of your energy needs to be focused on uncovering and honouring this person. The clearer you are as to the true you, the clearer your path, and the easier it is to spot the parts that are not true, i.e. the other you. The aspect of cancer that's important in this regard is the space and time it gives you to be you.

The pace of life in the West is extraordinarily hectic. Most of our days are spent working or catching up with things we have to do. There is little time to sit in silence and connect with truth. And even when we do have time, often the other you stops us from doing so (remember my feelings at the suggestion of a bath in the last chapter).

Part of cancer's power is its ability to create space where previously none existed. For me space came when, on the day of diagnosis, I stopped being a workaholic—something that, before then, had seemed impossible. Until cancer I spent virtually all of my child-free time working, or involved in community or other activities. As a result I had no free time and—this is why the other me did it—no time to connect with my truth.

Cancer connects us with a fundamental truth—that we are mortal and that we can, at any time, die—and with this truth comes clarity and perspective. We see what is real and what is illusion, i.e. what needs to stay and what can go, and from this space emerges. I didn't stop working when I had cancer—ceasing to be a workaholic and slowing down, especially around the operation and during chemotherapy, was enough for me—but taking time off work may be exactly what you need. Use this time to reconnect with the true you. This is your time—more so now than at any other point in your life—and you need to make the most of it.

Cancer has come to connect you with truth. To show you who you are—the true you—and who you are not—the other you—and to set out a path to follow. In the beginning you can stay on the path simply by acknowledging the issues that cancer raises and by dealing with them tirelessly and ceaselessly. The most difficult part comes later, i.e. when you no longer have cancer to light the way. I don't want to scare you with that statement. Given that you are in the middle of possibly the worst time in your life, the last thing you need is me telling you things will get harder. So I need to make it clear: I'm not saying this. It's not life that will get more difficult but staying on the path—and these two things are not the same at all.

The most difficult part of my cancer was the time following chemotherapy. Chemotherapy marked the end of my treatment and took place between July and October 2001. The worst part of all was the first quarter of 2002. By then I'd recovered from chemotherapy's immediate effects and was thinking forward to the rest of my life. Thinking this should have been a good time for me is looking at cancer through the eyes of the other you. From that perspective cancer is bad and no cancer is good, but from my perspective—that of my true you—cancer is truth, and without cancer there was the possibility of illusion and falling back. Thus, without cancer for the first time in almost a year, I was scared. I was afraid I would lose myself as I'd done when I let the know-it-alls get to me, and it was a very dark time.

Looking back I wasn't in any real danger. The point of no return had passed some months before when I'd talked to my parents. But it did feel dangerous and, as I see it now, it needed to. It was essential during that time that I stayed focused on my path, or rather that I stayed focused on finding my path given that it was lost from view. The fear was a way of maintaining that focus. The path had not disappeared but I could not, at first, see it on my own. I equate this with following tracks in the African bush. Initially I was led by an experienced guide, the cancer, and if I paid attention to what was shown to me the path was clear. When the guide left me at the end of chemotherapy, I was not used to seeing the path for myself and lost sight of it. I rediscovered it because I never stopped looking for it and had faith that I would find it again, as well as fear that I would not. I saw the path clearly when, around Easter 2002, I decided to sell my house and write this book.

I can remember little about the months at the beginning of 2002 other than the darkness of them and, despite what I said above, I don't remember having faith that I would find my path, only fear that I would not. So if it was not faith that brought me back to my path, what did? I think it was faith but of a different kind: a faith in myself that developed unknowingly alongside the cancer. I'm not sure when the faith started to grow but it was already visible on the day of diagnosis. When I blurted, "only if I want one," in response to, "you'll have to have an operation," that showed faith in myself. However, as I said before, my statement was out before I knew it. It's only later that my faith grew to such a degree that I was aware of it and could use it consciously. Key factors in this development were the 'run-ins' I had with my doctors.

I spent a lot of time with my lump—an hour or more each day cradling it in my hand—and as a result I knew it well. I was aware, therefore, that it was growing very quickly but also that it changed shape: sometimes it was spherical and at other times more like a flying saucer. I asked my regular doctor why this was; he didn't know but referred me to my surgeon. My surgeon's response was this: "It's not happening. It's not growing and it's not changing shape." It was then that I knew I had to change surgeons. I could not allow this person, someone who had no respect for me and no belief in me, to operate on me.

Even now, when faced with something that contradicts my own experience, I tend to believe what is being shown to me rather than what I know to be true. This doesn't happen as much as it used to, but it's still my default reaction to certain situations—and yet with cancer this reaction disappeared completely. I knew the lump was growing and changing shape, and nothing the surgeon said would make me believe otherwise. Cancer connected me with my truth like nothing else before or since and with it I was invincible.

Yesterday I sent an e-mail to a friend. The subject was vulnerability and, in particular, the way in which we are open to manipulation by others. In writing the e-mail I came to realise something: that only via the other you can we be manipulated. Thinking about the first three months of 2002 in these terms, this was a dark time for me because I had nothing concrete with which to access the true me, i.e. the cancer was gone. And, in the absence of this, there was an opening for the other me to take control and, via manipulation, for others to take control of me. It is this, in hindsight, I was afraid of.

Most of us do not set out to manipulate others but, unconsciously, this is what we do. When being the other you we avoid truth and manipulate others to stop truth being revealed. When I spoke to my surgeon about the changing shape of my lump, his response—his other you response—was to tell me this wasn't happening. Because I was in touch with my truth—quite literally, the lump being the physical manifestation of my truth—I could not be manipulated by him. I saw his behaviour for what it was—a sign that he was not the right surgeon for me—and swapped surgeons.

I don't know why the surgeon said what he did, but he was wrong to do so. The lump was changing shape and that's what breast lumps do. (I later read that breast lumps respond to phases in a woman's menstrual cycle, switching between the shape of a boiled egg—my sphere—and a fried egg—my flying saucer). The surgeon's reaction was, therefore, hiding something and I can only postulate what this might have been. Here are some possibilities (the real reason may have been completely different): he saw me as a troublemaker and wanted to shut me up; as a Consultant, he believed he knew everything and he'd not heard of lumps changing shape, therefore my lump could not have changed shape; he was running behind and didn't have time to talk; or he wanted to reassure me that all was well. However honourable or dishonourable his motives, I was right not to be drawn by his other-you behaviour—and this is *always* true. Following the path of the other you—yours or someone else's—can only ever be a detour on the path to truth.

I saw my first oncologist after my mastectomy. Based on the analysis of my lump he set out a treatment plan: a course of chemotherapy followed by hormone treatment.

Needing time to gather my thoughts, I took time out and went back to see him a week later. When we ran through the proposed treatment it now included radiotherapy. I was shocked and taken aback. "Why has the treatment plan changed?"

"It hasn't. I said last time you'd need radiotherapy."

He didn't. I know he didn't. However difficult a time it was for me, I know what was said. Leaving the room with a breast-care nurse, I asked to see another oncologist. This doctor took offence at me seeing an acupuncturist, in his eyes an unproven treatment, and for questioning his suggested approach. He was angry and aggressive and, therefore, also not right for me.

It's interesting for me to see how strong my resolve was back then. I had no qualms saying, "this doctor is not right for me," not once but three times, and asking for another. Writing about my experiences has also given me access to the feelings I had when making these decisions. At no time was I motivated by my intellect. My mind didn't tell me the doctors were wrong for me, it was my body, and my strength of feeling was such that I could not have allowed them to treat me. I could not act against what I knew to be true. It's easy to look at my experiences and think: "How unlucky!" In fact, the opposite is true. These encounters gave me the opportunity to experience my truth and to practice acting on it, and after a lifetime of hiding my truth this is something I very much needed to do.

The letter I sent to the third oncologist before meeting him shows not only that I have been true in reporting my experience of cancer—not that you had any doubts, I hope—but also how important it is to be true. The power of the letter comes, I believe, from acknowledging that I may have had a part to play in my experiences with the previous doctors, and from being clear about what it is I wanted from him.

> *Tuesday, 26 June 2001*
> *Dear Dr...*
> *I am coming to see you at your clinic...and am writing this letter in preparation for this meeting. I want the consultation to go as well as possible and hope that this letter will facilitate this. My breast-care nurse...suggested this approach after my last meeting with an oncologist and I very much feel that this is the right way forward.*
>
> *I don't know how most people relate to breast cancer, nor how they relate to their Doctors and other health-care professionals, but I am very clear what cancer means to me and the relationship I want/need with you and your colleagues. I just hope that I can put this into words that convey this to you.*
>
> *The only bad thing about cancer is that it threatens my life—and that's why I need your help. The thing is this aspect of the cancer seems so small and almost irrelevant compared with everything else it has given me. I don't want to die but when I think about death I have to hold that threat up against what life was like before I had cancer—I was dead already. I was cut-off, closed down, out of touch—if anything cancer has given me my life back. Cancer has allowed me to feel full of life again, joyous, hopeful, excited, bursting at the seams with energy. That is not how I felt before I had cancer—far from it—and I don't want to go back there. Refusing a planned operation at the end of March was largely about this—living that close to the edge was what I needed to uncover the roots of my problems and begin to deal with them.*
>
> *Where I am now is that I feel I need to have further treatment (I had a mastectomy at the end of April)—mainly because I can't see an end to this stage of my life/the cancer until I've done this.*

Having further treatment will enable me to close the chapter and move on. But in order to do this I need a Doctor I feel I can trust, unfortunately not something I have found in the oncology department at the[18]...(and this letter aims to alleviate my part in any communication difficulties which could prevent the development of such trust and understanding).

As a result of my experiences talking to two oncologists, a chemotherapy nurse, a radiotherapy nurse and my breast-care nurse...as well as Breast Cancer Care and an oncologist in Canada (the sister of a friend), I know that in order for me to be able to trust a doctor I need them to be consistent, open and honest, respectful of my views and prepared to answer my questions (with don't know being a perfectly acceptable answer). I've had this speaking to the Canadian oncologist but I need this here too. I can't put my life in the hands of someone I don't trust, I'd rather put faith in myself and God.

If I'm to go forward with chemotherapy and other treatments I need to be able to embrace these, to welcome them with open arms, knowing what I may have to face. In order for me to do this I need to be able to understand them and their possible benefits and side effects. As a result it would be helpful if we could talk about the following[19]...

I realise it may be an unusual step to contact you in this way and hope that you will understand my reasons for doing so. I very much look forward to meeting you...

Best Wishes

Lesley Moore

The letter had the desired effect and I found an oncologist I could communicate with and trust. On the basis of my Nottingham Prognostic Index (NPI), he recommended chemotherapy. The NPI uses three factors to predict survival: size of lump, cancer grade and lymph node stage. My NPI was 4.76 giving me a 51% chance of surviving ten years[20]. It was the grade of my cancer that contributed most to this value. It was estimated that, with chemotherapy, the likelihood of survival over ten years would increase from 51% to 75%.

From the letter, you know how I felt: that to move past that phase of my life and cancer, I had to have further treatment. What finally persuaded me to have chemotherapy was something quite different. I watched the film *Shakespeare in Love* and thought, "a love like that is worth living for". In the end, that's what did it. I needed a doctor I could trust, I needed to understand the treatment, its benefits and side effects, but I said yes to further treatment on the basis of love. Very fitting for a cancer diagnosed on Valentine's Day and that was, from the beginning, all about love.

59

And that's how to deal with proposed cancer treatments: get the information you need to make an informed decision, but let the true you lead you through. In that way you can satisfy your rational side (and shut it up) and at the same time satisfy (and shut up) those around you. When it comes to uncovering and honouring the true you, other people aren't much help; more often than not they're a hindrance. So caught up are they in the world of the other you, they fail to see the truth.

My mind is taken back to the mastectomy. I took the decision to go ahead with it less than 24 hours before it was due, so had little time to let people know. One of the few people I told in advance of the operation was my sister. I asked if she could look after my son while I was in hospital—she did—and also that she keep the operation secret from our parents—she did that too. From speaking to her later I know this involved lying to them, and so was not an easy thing for her to do. I'm grateful to her for this and consider that, of all the things she has done for me, this is the most important. If I think of my sister's love, it's this I remember. When I asked my sister not to tell my mum and dad about the operation I didn't know why this was necessary, but I felt very strongly—i.e. my body told me—that it had to be this way. It was only the day after the mastectomy that I understood.

I had my operation early in the day and was the first to be operated on by my surgeon. It was probably scheduled that way to prevent me hanging around and changing my mind. Given the size of my lump, the high grade of the cancer and the time since diagnosis (eleven weeks), both the surgeon and the breast-care nurse were keen for me to have the operation without further delay. Both had invested lots of time in me and were keen to see me jump through the hoop. But that sounds flippant and I don't mean it to be. It was that way, but what's missing from my statement is an appreciation of what they did for me and how this was, in the case of the surgeon at least, above and beyond the call of duty.

The breast-care nurse system is a good one. At the time of diagnosis you are assigned a nurse who guides you through the process. If you need comfort, you can get it from the breast-care nurse. If you need information, she (I didn't meet a male one) will get it for you. Her job is to support and care for you and to give you what you need. My breast-care nurse didn't understand where I was coming from with cancer—she did try—but that didn't stop her doing her job and doing it well. She did everything I asked, e.g. found papers on infertility following chemotherapy, and arranged the transfers between doctors and hospitals.

It was different with the surgeon, the second one. It wasn't his job to talk about my feelings or to try to understand me but that's exactly what he did, on one occasion meeting with me outside his regular time for patient consultation. The meeting took place soon after I was assigned to his care. It was held in one of the hospital's more cosy rooms, near to where the breast-care nurses had their offices. I sat in what passed in the hospital for a comfy chair and the surgeon and the breast-care nurse sat opposite. I remember him in a chair that was taller than mine, but that probably says more about my emotional state than the reality of the situation. The entrance to the room was to my right and to my left was a large window. It was just before the first day of spring and the room was filled with the sun's warmth and light. I can't remember why we met. It was probably to continue a conversation that started during my first appointment with him, but of that first meeting I have no memory.

Our meeting in the cosy room could be judged, by some, as unsuccessful and a waste of time. It lasted around an hour and by the end of it nothing had been resolved. The surgeon wanted me to have a mastectomy but I could not say yes. I explained, as best I could, my feelings about the cancer and my fears about going forward without it, but it was only a month after the diagnosis and back then I didn't have the words. I fumbled and stumbled around the issues saying things such as, "death doesn't seem as bad as the other options", and my fragmented and incomplete explanations did little to help his understanding. But that is not important. What matters is that the surgeon made time to listen and tried to understand, and because of this I trusted and respected him. At the end of the meeting I was frustrated that I could not put into words my feelings, but my feelings towards him were only positive. As a result, when, about five or six weeks later, I decided to go ahead with the mastectomy, I did so safe in the knowledge that he was performing the operation and that he would look after me as best he could. From my perspective, the meeting in the cosy room was a resounding success.

A mastectomy is not like other operations. Because it involves the loss of a breast, there is an extreme brutality to it. When my breast-care nurse showed me pictures of women who had undergone mastectomies, what struck me is how brutal and primitive it is: "Here we are in the 21st Century and yet the best the medical profession can offer is to cut off my breast with a knife!" They do this because breast cancer is a killer and because a mastectomy is an effective treatment—but that doesn't make it easier to countenance. Indeed, so difficult is it to face that most women go ahead with the operation without seeing what will happen to them. My breast-care nurse was surprised when I asked to see pictures of mastectomies—most women do not—and checked at least twice that this was, in fact, what I wanted. I needed to see those pictures. I needed to understand what a mastectomy involved so that I could come to terms with it and embrace it. When I went down to the operating theatre I was fully conscious. The nurse tried to give me a pre-op (a drug to make me drowsy) but I refused. "I want to know what I'm doing," I said. "I want to be in control and know I've not been coerced into this." I went into the operation eyes wide open; for me it had to be that way.

Being ready to embrace the operation didn't happen by chance. As I said in Chapter 4, it's the "huge effort that goes into being ready that it's important to grasp and appreciate". A week after the diagnosis I had a dream that a doctor was trying to rape me. This was, I'm sure, a response to the proposed mastectomy and a visual representation of the rape archetype. In her book, *Women's Bodies Women's Wisdom*, Dr Christiane Northrup has the following to say about archetypes: "Archetypes are psychological and emotion patterns that influence us unconsciously until we become aware of their power. Archetypes are universal ideas, images and patterns of thought that we all share in our subconscious. Though the concept of archetypes may at first seem elusive, these unconscious patterns of thought and behaviour have a very real effect on our bodies and emotions. When a woman feels that she is forced to participate in an activity, her body, mind and spirit are at risk of harm. When she unwittingly participates in a pattern of self-abuse and abuse from others, she is acting under the influence of what in energy medicine is called the 'rape' archetype...The 'rape' archetype may [also] occur when a woman participates in her own violation."

Whatever the medical need and associated benefits, a mastectomy *is* a violation. It's no surprise, therefore, that women find it hard to approach willingly. Taking time to ensure that I had a good relationship with a caring doctor was integral to me allowing myself to be violated in this way and not suffering unduly because of it. So, my preparation for the mastectomy was threefold: getting the information I needed, e.g. the post-operative pictures; finding a surgeon I could trust; and saying goodbye to my breast. I did the last of these the evening before the mastectomy.

As on so many occasions I sat with my breast cradled in my hand, but this was to be the last time. I can't remember the thoughts in my head or the emotions that surfaced, but I can remember the tears — so many tears — and remembering that time now the tears have come again. But they are not, as you may think, for the loss of my breast, but for the nature of that moment and in particular for its humanity. That evening was one of the rare times — perhaps the only time — I experienced cancer from a purely human perspective. To make myself ready for the operation I intuitively lay aside all that I knew about cancer — its purpose, its power and its truth — and allowed myself to be only with its physicality. On that night cancer meant loss of a breast and I grieved for that loss as I should.

And so it was that, the day after the mastectomy, I took off my pyjama top and looked into the mirror, saw the space where my breast had been and felt nothing. Not because I was numb or unable to access my emotions, but because there was nothing to feel. I've not shed a tear for the loss of my breast since the night before the operation; sometimes I've tried to be upset, wondering whether I was blocking the upset, but the upset is not there. And standing in the hospital bathroom, as I raised my eyes from the bandage taped to my skin to look at myself as a whole, the reason for not telling my parents became clear. I needed to know how *I* felt before *they* told me. So when they rushed to my side following my 'phone call, thrilled that I'd finally done what the doctors had recommended and that they so desperately wanted, I was able to say in response to: "It must be terrible".

"It's not like that at all."

I had my mastectomy eleven weeks after the initial diagnosis. In that time the lump had grown from the size of a pea to that of a tangerine. My cancer was the most aggressive form and the fear was that it had spread. When the results showed the cancer had been contained in my breast, my surgeon—not a man known for his colloquialisms—said: "I'm gob-smacked!"

Was I gob-smacked? No. To me it made perfect sense. I had the operation on the advice of my body the day after it said: "We can't hold this off much longer." As well as conveying the importance of swift action, this statement also revealed I had been in safe hands. My body gave me cancer to put me in touch with the true me, and it protected me while I established and strengthened that connection.

60

And so we've reached the end of the book, or at least the final chapter. My story has been told. I've shared my wisdom with you. And now it's up to you. Essentially, you are the same person as the one who picked up this book: you have cancer and you have to deal with it. But having read my story you can now view it differently. Cancer can be a terrible thing, a cruel twist of fate and a living nightmare, or it can be the path back to you. It's up to you which one you choose.

The first, more common, path is well known to you and those around you, and is easier to find. So clearly is it mapped and so full of travellers, most find themselves on it without a second thought. It is, so most would have you believe, the only path. And yet there is another. Aside from the number of companions there is little, in the beginning, to separate and distinguish the paths. Defined as they are by the physicality of cancer, both the landscape and the landmarks are the same. All that the less common path offers is a different point of view.

For those on the traditional path the journey is a dark one, overshadowed by the fear of death. Landmarks loom ahead as vast grey monuments and the landscape, full of strange sights and hidden whispers, is to be passed with speed. Travelling along the alternate route the journey is experienced differently. Clutching in one hand a divine light, those opting for this path set out on a pilgrimage. Safe in the knowledge that all is well, landmarks are seen not only in terms of their scale, but also for their subtlety and tone. And while taking care to stay on the path, those on it are able to scan the landscape in search of its treasures.

Only as cancer ends do the paths diverge. Those who survive the journey find that one path leads back to the land before cancer and the other into the unknown. She who takes the common path finds herself in familiar territory; cancer was, thankfully, just a diversion from the previous path. But what of the other travellers? Those who opted for the different route?

There is much to be explored.

If you opt for the path I took, I'm glad. There is one more thing I can offer to help you on your journey. There will be times when you lose your way and find yourself back on the common path. Do not despair, for this is bound to happen. I've prepared a list of other-you thoughts and emotions that arise at such times, along with the true-you response. These will help you shift back to your chosen path.

Whichever path you take I wish you good health and good speed. May God—the universal positive energy that is both eternal and infinite—be with you on your journey.

Other-You Thoughts and Emotions
True-You Response

My life was going well. Cancer messed things up.
I was not living my truth. Cancer came to reveal my true self.

Life is unfair.
Through the eyes of the true you, life is generous beyond measure. What I learn in this life my soul carries for eternity.

Why me?
There is a reason why. If I ask my body why, then I will know.

My body has gone wrong.
My body is showing me how far I have strayed from my path.

I feel helpless. I don't know where to turn.
I have faith in myself and my body. What I need for my journey will be given.

I am angry. I am afraid. I am upset. I am panicked.
Emotion is a communication from my body. It reveals a part of the other me. If I look at emotion with my body, I will find a path back to truth.

There is so much to cope with.
Cancer has revealed internal struggles that were previously hidden. With cancer I can put an end to these once and for all.

Life won't be the same.
No longer will I be controlled and caged by the other me.

I don't know how to fight cancer.
The fight against cancer is a fight against the other me. If I listen to my body, the true me will show me the way.

I'm not sure which treatment to have.
Cancer has both a spiritual and a physical dimension. I must pay attention to both, using my body and my intellect to map the way forward.

I'm scared I won't find the right path.
There is no right path. There is only my *path. If I listen to my body, my path will become clear.*

I might die. I don't want to die.
Coming to terms with death is essential for a full and fulfilling life.

The doctor has told me I am going to die.
As the other me dies, the true me is born again. The true me is eternal and divine.

Endpiece

I'll leave you with my wishes for my end. In other words, what I'd like to happen when I die. I want to achieve a rainbow body as described in *The Tibetan Book of Living and Dying*[21].

It is possible for some people, normally accomplished Buddhist practitioners but for Westerners also, to "bring their lives to an extraordinary and triumphant end. As they die they enable their body to be reabsorbed back into the light essence of the light elements that created it, and consequently their material body dissolves into light and disappears completely. This process is known as the 'rainbow body' or 'body of light' because the dissolution is often accompanied by spontaneous manifestations of light and rainbows..."

Ancient writings distinguish "different categories of this amazing otherworldly phenomenon, for at one time, if at least not normal, it was reasonably frequent". If I achieve a rainbow body and someone is around to see it and maybe even record it, I hope it will be enough to stop in your tracks those of you for whom cancer and my story were not enough.

And finally, my epitaph:

When you remember me
Remember we are the same

Bibliography

Ancient Wisdom, Modern World, Ethics for the New Millennium, Tenzin Gyatso, His Holiness the Dalai Lama, Abacus, London, 2001, ISBN 0316858633

Buddhism for Today and Tomorrow, Sangharakshita, Windhorse Publications, Birmingham, 1996, ISBN 0904766837

Cave in the Snow, Vicki Mackenzie, Bloomsbury, London, 1999, ISBN 0747543895

Chambers English Dictionary, 7th Edition, W&R Chambers Ltd, Edinburgh, 1990, ISBN 0550102507

Health Statistics Quarterly 21, *Table 6.1 Deaths: Age and Sex, Numbers and Rates, 1976 onwards (England and Wales)*, National Statistics website, http:/www.statistics.gov.uk/STATBASE/Expodata/Spreadsheets/D7629.xls

Ingenious Pain, Andrew Miller, Sceptre, London, 1998, ISBN 0340682086

Journeys (with a Cancer), Jenny Cole, Pawprints, London, 1995, ISBN 0952533847

Meeting Jesus Again for the First Time: The Historical Jesus and the Heart of Contemporary Faith, Marcus Borg, 1995, Harper, San Francisco, ISBN 0060609176

Quantum Healing: Exploring the Frontiers of Mind/Body Medicine, Deepak Chopra, Bantam, London, 1989, ISBN 0553348698

Stories of the Celtic Soul Friends, Edward Sellner, Paulist Press, Mahwah, New Jersey, 2004, ISBN 0809141116

The Tibetan Book of Living and Dying, A Spiritual Classic from One of the Foremost Interpreters of Tibetan Buddhism to the West, Sogyal Rinpoche, Rider & Co, London, 2002, ISBN 0712615695

Women Who Run with the Wolves: Myths and Stories of the Wild Woman Archetype, Clarissa Pinkola Estés, Rider, London, 1998 Edition, ISBN 071267134X

Women's Bodies Women's Wisdom, Dr Christiane Northrup, 2001 edition, Piatkus, London, ISBN 0749919256

Endnotes

[1] Unless otherwise stated all definitions are taken from Chambers English Dictionary, 7th Edition.

[2] More than one in three people will be diagnosed with a cancer during their lifetime and one in four will die from cancer. *Cancer Facts and Figures*, Cancer Research UK, downloaded from http://www.cancerresearchuk.org/ aboutcancer/statistics/ on 10/5/05.

[3] Figures for 2001, *Breast Cancer Facts and Statistics*, downloaded from the Breast Cancer Care website 8/1/04.

[4] Estimated new cancer deaths and cases for 2005, *SEER Cancer Statistic Review 1975-2002*, National Cancer Institute. Available on the internet.

[5] 75% to 80% of breast cancer detected in Canada through breast cancer screening is invasive. *Questions and Answers on Breast Cancer*, 1998, ISBN 092999116921X, Canadian Breast Cancer Care Initiative.

[6] The text between note 5 and 6 is paraphrased from text in the booklet *Treating Breast Cancer* (September 2000 version), ISBN 1870577019, Breast Cancer Care.

[7] *Ibid* for this sentence. *Ibid* is Latin and means the same reference as the last one.

[8] *Clinical Practice Guidelines for the Care and Treatment of Breast Cancer*, Supplement to the Canadian Medical Association Journal, February 10, 1998; 158 (3 Suppl).

[9] A chakra is a centre of spiritual power in the body. There are seven chakras: root or base, naval, solar plexus, heart, throat, brow (the third eye) and crown.

[10] Pulses are the energy signatures of the organs in the body. Acupuncturists use pulses to assess the health of a patient and to determine and monitor treatments.

[11] Odds of winning the UK lottery jackpot with one ticket are 1 in 13,983,816, i.e. the probability of matching six balls out of a possible 49 is $6/49 \times 5/48 \times 4/47 \times 3/46 \times 2/45 \times 1/44 = 1/13,983,816$. Likelihood of death for a 30-year-old woman is 1 in 2,273 per annum. Thus, she is 6,152.14 times more likely to die in any given year than win the lottery if she buys one ticket that year (i.e. $13,983,816/2,273 = 6,152.14$). She would need to buy at least 6,153 tickets in a year (118.33 per week) for her chance of winning the lottery to exceed her chance of dying. Assuming she buys 119 tickets per week, the cost would be £6,188 (i.e. $119 \times 52 \times £1$).

[12] Assuming her partner is in the same age group the odds of him dying are 1 in 1,064 per annum. Thus it is 13,142.68 times more likely that he will die in any given year than the family win the lottery if the woman buys one ticket that year (i.e. $13,983,816/1,064 = 13,142.68$). She would need to buy at least 13,143 tickets in a year (252.75 per week) to ensure that her chance of winning the lottery exceeds his chance of dying. To ensure the odds of her winning the lottery exceed the odds of her *or* her partner dying, she

would need to buy 372 tickets per week (i.e. 119 for her + 253 for him = 372). The cost of these tickets would be £19,344 (i.e. 372 x 52 x £1).

[13] 100 thoughts a day is 36,500 a year (100 x 365 = 36,500). This level of thoughts over 28 years is 1,022,000 thoughts (36,500 x 28 = 1,022,000).

[14] The idea of the sacred as an experiential reality is taken from *Stories of Celtic Soul Friends* by Edward Sellner, who in turn borrowed it from *Meeting Jesus Again for the First Time* by Marcus Borg.

[15] Definitions downloaded on 15/5/04 from http://deadlysins. com/

[16] The phrase "teach and communicate his vision" is taken from *Buddhism for Today and Tomorrow* by Sangharakshita.

[17] *ibid* for "of its very nature, incommunicable."

[18] The letter was written to a Doctor around 75 miles away from my home and the hospital where I had my mastectomy.

[19] What followed was a list of questions concerning chemotherapy and radiotherapy. It is not appropriate to include these here.

[20] Survival rates are taken from RW Blamey, *The Design and Clinical Use of the Nottingham Prognostic Index in Breast Cancer*, The Breast 1996, 156-7.
NPI = Size (in cm) x 0.2 + Grade (I to III) + Stage (1 to 3)

My lump was 3.8 cm. My cancer was Grade III and the Stage was 1 (no lymph node involvement). The relationship between NPI and 10 year survival (NPI: 10 year survival) is: ≤2.4: 94%; ≤3.4: 83%; ≤4.4: 70%; <5.4: 51%; >5.4: 19%. Lymph node stages are: 1 no nodal involvement; 2 involvement of up to three low axillary nodes OR an internal mammary node (for medical tumours); 3 involvement of four or more low axillary nodes and/or the apical node, or any low axillary node and internal mammary node simultaneously.

[21] This idea is taken from the book *Cave in the Snow* by Vicki Mackenzie, which tells the story of Tenzin Palmo a western woman who became a Buddhist nun. The book includes this quote from *The Tibetan Book of Living and Dying* by Sogyal Rinpoche.

Made in the USA